IEP Goal Writing for Speech-Language Pathologists

Utilizing State Standards

IEP Goal Writing for Speech-Language Pathologists

Utilizing State Standards

Lydia Kopel, EdS, CCC-SLP
Elissa Kilduff, MA, CCC-SLP

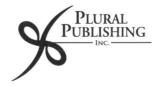
PLURAL
PUBLISHING
INC.

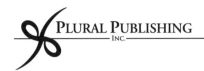

5521 Ruffin Road
San Diego, CA 92123

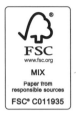

e-mail: info@pluralpublishing.com
Website: http://www.pluralpublishing.com

Typeset in 12/16 Palatino by Flanagan's Publishing Services, Inc.
Printed in the United States of America by McNaughton & Gunn, Inc.
20 19 18 17   3 4 5 6

Library of Congress Cataloging-in-Publication Data

Names: Kopel, Lydia, author. | Kilduff, Elissa, author.
Title: IEP goal writing for speech-language pathologists utilizing state
   standards / Lydia Kopel, Elissa Kilduff.
Description: San Diego, CA : Plural Publishing, Inc, [2016] | Includes
   bibliographical references and index.
Identifiers: LCCN 2015046758 | ISBN 9781597569415 | ISBN 1597569410
Subjects: | MESH: Language Disorders—rehabilitation | Speech-Language
   Pathology—methods | Education—standards | Goals | Child | Adolescent |
   United States
Classification: LCC RC428 | NLM WL 340.2 | DDC 616.85/50071—dc23
LC record available at http://lccn.loc.gov/2015046758

Contents

Preface

As speech-language pathologists (SLPs), we have a responsibility to support the state standards. In order for students to be successful with the standards, they must have mastered specific speech-language skills. There are three objectives of this book. First, to familiarize the SLP with specific Early Learning Standards and Common Core State Standards (CCSS) and the speech-language skills needed to be successful with these standards. The second objective is to outline prerequisite speech-language skills and steps to mastering those skills. The third objective, through a step-by-step process, is to write defensible IEP goals that are related to the standards.

The information and process provided in this book are based on research, fifty years of combined experience as school-based SLPs and administrators, and reviewing Individualized Education Programs (IEPs) from all over the country. The authors developed this book as a result of reading hundreds of IEPs that had goals and objectives that were difficult to implement as written. This process has been field tested through a large metro school system with more than 175 SLPs.

OBJECTIVE 1: EARLY LEARNING STANDARDS AND COMMON CORE STATE STANDARDS AND ASSOCIATED PREREQUISITE SPEECH-LANGUAGE SKILLS

Early Learning Standards are the developmental building blocks for success in school. These are focused on in Chapter 1. These standards were developed using the Head Start Early Learning Outcomes Framework: Ages Birth to Five (Office of Head Start, 2015) and individual state's early learning standards for three and four year olds. They are divided into the areas of Communication and Literacy, Math, Science, Social Studies, Cognition, Approaches to Learning, and Social and Emotional.

The CCSS (National Governors Association Center for Best Practices [NGA Center] & Council of Chief State School Officers [CCSSO], 2010) requires a strong foundation of speech-language skills and these are the focus of Chapter 2. Standards have been pulled from all areas including English Language Arts, Literacy in History/Social Studies, Science, Technical Subjects, and Mathematics. The standards are organized by grade level. Within each grade level the standards are organized by Common Core area, numbers, as indicated in the CCSS, and specific prerequisite speech and language skill(s) for that standard.

The Early Learning Standards can easily be compared to the Early Learning Standards from each state. In addition, for those SLPs whose state or school system has not adopted the Common Core State Standards, these can be compared to their adopted standards. This process can assist SLPs in identifying target skills within those standards.

OBJECTIVE 2: PREREQUISITE SKILLS AND STEPS TO MASTERY

Chapter 3 consists of the speech-language skills that, in our experience, are the commonly addressed skills of intervention for students aged 3 years–21 years, with all levels of functioning. These skills are organized by the following speech-language areas: *Vocabulary, Questions, Summarize, Main idea and Details, Critical Thinking, Pragmatics, Syntax and Morphology,* and *Articulation and Phonological Processes.* Every speech and language skill has several prerequisite skills which have been outlined in Chapter 3. Each *Prerequisite Skill* then has corresponding *Steps to Mastery* that should be achieved in order to succeed with the state standards. The *Steps to Mastery* are a hierarchy of levels from easiest to most difficult that should be accomplished for mastery of each *Prerequisite Skill.*

OBJECTIVE 3: STEP-BY-STEP PROCESS TO WRITING IEP GOALS

Once the SLP has identified the curriculum areas and specific standards that a student is struggling with, the Early Learning Standards in Chapter 1 and/or the CCSS in Chapter 2 should be reviewed. These standards identify specific prerequisite speech and language skills the student may be lacking. Next, the SLP would look up the *Prerequisite Skills* in Chapter 3 to determine which corresponding *Steps to Mastery* the student requires. The SLP then writes the IEP goal for the final *Step to Mastery* that the student can reasonably achieve in the course of the IEP. The *Steps to Mastery* can be easily developed into IEP goals. The *Goal Writing Worksheet* and information in Chapter 4 will assist the SLP with this process. It will also provide the framework for writing defensible IEP goals. The components of this framework include ensuring that the goals are understandable, doable, measurable, and achievable. An example of the goal writing process is included below.

D.J., 5th Grader—Classroom teacher reports that D.J. is having trouble with main idea and supporting details.

- Identify the 5th-grade CCSS in Chapter 2 that align with the skills of main idea.

- Go to the Main Idea & Details section in Chapter 3 and look at all the *Prerequisite Skills*. The skills listed are:
  - Comprehending questions
  - Sequence
  - Main idea when stated
  - Important versus unimportant details
  - Infer/draw conclusions
  - Main idea and supporting details

- Decide where the student is currently functioning. In this case, D.J. can answer questions and sequence. That means he would start with "main idea when stated."

- Starting with "main idea when stated," look at all the *Steps to Mastery* under each of the subsequent *Prerequisite Skills*.

- Decide how many steps D.J. can reasonably achieve in the course of the IEP. In this case, it is believed that D.J.can get partway through the "main idea and supporting details" *Steps to Mastery*; up to "Identify ___#___ details that support a given main idea in a _____ (paragraph, story, poem, chapter, etc.)." Write the goal using the *Goal Writing Worksheet*.
  - D.J. will state three details that support a given main idea in a grade-level passage when read aloud to him in four out of five opportunities using data collection.

This book focuses on skills for mastery, not on activities. The activities will vary from student to student and need to reflect the Universal Design for Learning (i.e., using multiple means of representation, expression, and engagement) (Rose & Gravel, 2010).

The concentration of this book is spoken language (receptive language, and expressive language) and articulation. Reading and writing are addressed through highlighting the underpinning language skills of reading and writing standards. A student's ability and progress on a spoken language IEP goal should not be measured based on abilities with written language alone. If we take away the expectation of reading and writing, we can better measure if a student is struggling with comprehension versus basic reading, or the ability to formulate a cohesive thought versus the ability to write. According to *Roles and Responsibilities of Speech-Language Pathologists with Respect to Reading and Writing in Children and Adolescents* (ASHA, 2001), SLPs working in the school system are one member of a team with various areas of expertise. Spoken language should not be looked at in isolation but considered along with written language and addressed as a team. It is important for SLPs to consider how students are using basic language knowledge and skills for the reading and writing processes. However, as direct service providers, SLPs should focus intervention on the language skills that underlie and impact the ability to acquire reading and writing. The SLP can then collaborate with other professionals in the school who provide interventions related to written language. Written language materials are imperative as part of spoken language intervention. SLPs should not be working on listening comprehension in the absence of reading material or oral expression in the absence of writing.

This is not intended to be an exhaustive list of speech-language skills. It is intended to target the common skills that SLPs focus on in the school system. There are many other skills that can be addressed as goals on a student's IEP. The key to remember is that the goal must be understandable, doable, measureable, and achievable. Goals are an ending point, not a beginning point.

This book provides clear guidelines of quantifiable building blocks to achieve specific goals defined by the child's IEP. SLPs are instrumental in helping students develop speech and language skills essential for mastery of the standards. With a clear understanding of early learning standards, state standards, prerequisite skills, and steps to mastery, interventions will be successful to help students achieve their IEP goals and have success with the curriculum.

1

Early Learning Standards

Currently, no national Early Learning Standards have been developed. The Office of Head Start (2015) developed the Head Start Early Learning Outcomes Framework: Ages Birth to Five. This provides a research-based description of the progress children make in the development and learning of school readiness skills. It describes the developmental progression and the preschool outcomes, including specific indicators for children by age 5. The Framework was developed to help guide early learning programs in designing curriculum. Individual states utilized this Framework and additional resources to develop their own sets of Early Learning Standards. States organize their Early Learning Standards in various ways: one set of standards for birth through age 5; one set for ages 3 to 5; a set for 4 year olds; or a separate set for 3 and 4 year olds. The Early Learning Standards included in this book were based on the states using separate standards for both 3 and 4 year olds. The Head Start Framework and individual state standards were compared and selected based on comprehensiveness and clarity. The standards are organized into the following areas:

- Communication and Literacy

- Math

- Science

- Social Studies

- Cognition

- Approaches to Learning

- Social and Emotional

Each Early Learning Standard includes the area, state where it was derived, the standard, and the specific prerequisite speech and language skills that are required to develop that standard. The SLP will use this chapter to help identify the *Prerequisite Skills* a student is lacking. There are times when just pragmatics or syntax/morphology is indicated for the prerequisite speech-language skills. When this happens, it is referring to all pragmatic skills or all syntax and morphology skills. The next step is to proceed to Chapter 3 to locate the *Prerequisite Skills* and *Steps to Mastery*.

Any individual state's Early Learning Standards can be compared to standards in this chapter. This can assist SLPs in identifying prerequisite skills in their state's standards.

3 YEAR OLDS			
Area	**State**	**Early Learning Standard**	**Speech and Language Skills**
Communication and Literacy	Louisiana	Follows two-step directions.	Concepts
	Kansas	Uses frequently occurring nouns and verbs when speaking.	Nouns Verbs
	Kansas	Understands and uses some question words (i.e., interrogatives) (e.g., who, what, where, when, why, how).	Ask questions Answer questions
	Kansas	Uses some basic qualitative (e.g., wet/dry, hot/cold) and quantitative (e.g., more/less, empty/full) concepts to describe familiar people, places, things, and events.	Concepts Describe
	Kansas	Able to describe objects and actions depicted in pictures.	Describe
	Kansas	Provides a label when given a "child-friendly" definition of a familiar word (e.g., what is round and bounces: a ball).	Nouns Verbs Adjectives
	District of Columbia	Uses simple pronouns (e.g., I, me, you, mine, he, she).	Pronouns
	Rhode Island	Understands increasingly longer and complex sentences, including sentences with two or more phrases or ideas.	Syntax/morphology
	Rhode Island	Uses longer, more increasingly complex sentences, including complete four- to six-word sentences.	Syntax/morphology
	Kansas	With prompting and support, asks and answers simple questions about the story content.	Ask questions Answer questions
	Rhode Island	Begins to understand the sequence of a story.	Sequence
	Kansas	Uses pictures and illustrations to tell and retell parts of a story.	Retell

3 Year Olds *continued*

Area	State	Early Learning Standard	Speech and Language Skills
Communication and Literacy	Kansas	Retells some details of the text using pictures or props as a support.	Retell
	Louisiana	With prompting and support, talks about or draws a character, setting, event, or idea in a text read aloud.	Narrative elements
	Louisiana	Describes picture and/or dictates story to caretaker.	Describe
	Georgia	Describes activities and experiences using details.	Describe Supporting details
	Rhode Island	Demonstrates an understanding of the meaning of words by describing the use of familiar objects, talking about categories of objects, using several words to explain the same idea (i.e., synonyms), and relating words to their opposites.	Adjectives Describe Categorize Antonyms Synonyms
	Kansas	With prompting and support compares and contrasts the adventures and experiences of the characters to self (e.g., "I have a red cape just like Goldilocks!").	Compare/contrast
	Kansas	With prompting and support identifies similarities between two texts on the same topic (e.g., in illustrations, descriptions, or procedures).	Compare/contrast
	District of Columbia	Makes predictions and/or asks questions about the text by examining the title, cover, pictures.	Ask questions Predict
	Georgia	Responds to more complex questions with appropriate answers.	Answer questions
	Kansas	Begins to form regular plural nouns orally by adding /s/ or /es/ (e.g., dog, dogs; wish, wishes).	Nouns Regular plurals
	Kansas	Distinguishes among a few verbs describing the same general action (e.g., walk, march, strut, prance) by acting out the meanings.	Verbs Synonyms

3 Year Olds *continued*

Area	State	Early Learning Standard	Speech and Language Skills
Communication and Literacy	Georgia	Listens and understands new vocabulary from activities, stories and books.	Vocabulary
	District of Columbia	Begins to use some words that are not a part of everyday conversational speech but that are learned through books and personal experiences (e.g., gigantic, rapidly, frustrated, transportation, race, or jog).	Vocabulary
	Rhode Island	Determines, with modeling and support, the meanings of unknown words by asking questions or using contextual clues, such as pictures that accompany text.	Meaning from context Ask questions
	North Carolina	Uses more than one word for the same object and uses words for parts of object (e.g., dog, beagle, Rover; arm, leg).	Nouns Synonyms
	District of Columbia	Uses speech that is mostly intelligible to familiar and unfamiliar adults.	Articulation/ phonological processes
	Kansas	Differentiates between sounds that are the same and different (e.g., environmental sounds, animal sounds, phonemes).	Compare/contrast
	Kansas	Identifies two words that start with the same sound (e.g., ball and bat both start with the /b/ sound).	Concepts Compare/contrast
	North Carolina	With prompting and support, makes comments and asks questions related to the topic of discussion.	Ask questions Topic maintenance
	North Carolina	Uses sentences or questions to ask for things (people, actions, objects, pets) or gain information.	Ask questions Request help, information, clarification
	North Carolina	Communicates messages with expression, tone, and inflection appropriate to the situation.	Nonverbal cues

3 Year Olds *continued*

Area	State	Early Learning Standard	Speech and Language Skills
Communication and Literacy	Rhode Island	Demonstrates an understanding of nonverbal cues (e.g., eye contact, distance from partner, and facial expressions) and the ability to use them.	Nonverbal cues
	Rhode Island	Engages, with support and modeling, in conversations of at least three turns, with each exchange relating to and building upon what was said previously.	Responding Initiating conversation Topic maintenance
Math	Georgia	Labels objects using size words.	Concepts
	Georgia	Identifies and duplicates simple, repeating patterns.	Concepts Match Sequence
	Georgia	Follows simple directions which demonstrate an understanding of directionality, order, and position of objects.	Concepts
	Rhode Island	Names familiar two-dimensional shapes (circle, triangle, square, rectangle), regardless of their size or orientation.	Nouns
	District of Columbia	Sorts and classifies objects by one attribute into two or more groups (e.g., color, size, shape).	Adjectives Sort Categorize
	District of Columbia	Uses positional vocabulary (e.g., up/down, in/out, on/off, under) to identify and describe the location of an object.	Concepts Prepositions Describe
	Louisiana	Tells "how many" after counting a set of five or fewer items (e.g., fingers, blocks, crayons).	Concepts Answer questions
	Louisiana	Identifies an object or person as first.	Concepts
	Louisiana	Describes some measurable attributes (length and weight) of objects and materials (e.g. big/little, long/short, heavy/not heavy).	Concepts Describe

3 Year Olds *continued*

Area	State	Early Learning Standard	Speech and Language Skills
Math	Kansas	When shown a collection of up to three items, creates another collection of equal amounts, not necessarily by matching (precursor to subitizing).	Concepts
	Kansas	Identifies whether the number of objects in one group is more or less as compared to the number of objects in another group up to five.	Concepts Compare/contrast
	North Carolina	Shows understanding that adding objects to a group will make a bigger group, and taking away objects will make a smaller group.	Comparatives/ superlatives
	Rhode Island	Uses comparative language (e.g., "shortest," "heavier," "biggest").	Comparatives/ superlatives
	Louisiana	Compares the size or weight of more than two objects and describes which one is longer/taller/ shorter/heavier/lighter.	Concepts Comparatives/ superlatives Compare/contrast
	Kansas	Analyzes and compares shapes in different sizes and orientations and uses informal language to describe their similarities, difference and part (e.g., number of sides and corners) and other attributes (e.g., having sides of equal length).	Concepts Describe Compare/contrast
Science	Georgia	Identifies and describes the functions of a few body parts.	Describe
	Louisiana	Describes what they see, hear, and are able to touch in the environment and groups materials/ objects according to observed features.	Describe Categorize
	Louisiana	Sorts living creatures and plants according to at least one characteristic (e.g., size, four-legged animals, hard/soft, etc.).	Sort Categorize
	Rhode Island	Uses observable characteristics to describe and categorize physical objects and materials based on differences or similarities.	Describe Categorize Compare/contrast

3 Year Olds *continued*

Area	State	Early Learning Standard	Speech and Language Skills
Science	Tennessee	Understands sequencing and time in relation to daily routines.	Concepts Sequence
	Kansas	Acquires and uses basic vocabulary for plants, animals and humans (e.g., some names of parts, characteristics).	Vocabulary
	Tennessee	Begins to describe and identify the similarities, categories, and different structures of familiar plants and animals.	Describe Categorize Compare/contrast
	District of Columbia	Asks more detailed questions including the relationship between two things or cause and effect relationships.	Ask questions Compare/contrast Cause/effect
	District of Columbia	Identifies a problem and, with adult assistance designs a solution (e.g., device or process) to address that problem.	Problem solve
	Rhode Island	Describes how living things change over time.	Describe Sequence Concepts
	District of Columbia	Compares and contrasts basic features of living things (e.g., body parts and their uses) between and across groups.	Compare/contrast
	District of Columbia	Compares and contrasts attributes of common materials related to their function (e.g., flexibility, transparency, strength).	Adjectives Compare/contrast
	Louisiana	With prompting and support, talks about observations and results of simple experiments verbally and/or through drawings or graphs.	Describe Cause/effect
	Rhode Island	Explores cause-and-effect relationships by intentionally varying the action to change the reaction (e.g., changing the size and/or orientation of blocks used when attempting to build a tall structure that doesn't fall down).	Cause/effect

3 Year Olds *continued*

Area	State	Early Learning Standard	Speech and Language Skills
Science	Louisiana	With prompting and support, talks about cause and effect relationships that are not immediately observable (e.g., that a plant wilted because it was not watered).	Cause/effect
	Louisiana	Asks why and how questions and offers ideas about living creatures, objects, materials, and changes they see, hear and/or feel.	Ask questions
	Louisiana	With prompting and support, talks about the meaning of words that are related to the scientific process (e.g., "observation," "experiment").	Vocabulary
	Louisiana	With prompting and support, observes and describes properties of objects and materials, and how objects and materials can be combined or can change from one form to another (e.g., ice melting to a liquid).	Describe Cause/effect
	Louisiana	Describes common weather conditions of the current season and how they compare to other seasons where they live (e.g., summer is hot, winter is cooler).	Describe Compare/contrast
	Louisiana	Names the types of clothing needed for different seasons.	Nouns Categorize
	Rhode Island	Makes simple predictions and plans to carry out investigations.	Predict
Social Studies	District of Columbia	Demonstrates awareness of a variety of jobs in the community and the work associated with them through conversation and/or play.	Nouns Verbs
	Kansas	Uses words to indicate direction.	Concepts Prepositions
	Georgia	Explains traditions and cultural celebrations of his/her own family.	Describe
	Georgia	Asks simple questions about others' cultures.	Ask questions

3 Year Olds *continued*

Area	State	Early Learning Standard	Speech and Language Skills
Social Studies	District of Columbia	Demonstrates an understanding of self as part of a family (e.g., parents, grandparents, siblings, caregivers).	Vocabulary
	Louisiana	Identifies the characteristics of one's own home.	Nouns Adjectives
	Louisiana	Describes familiar places such as the home, center/family day home, etc.	Describe
	Louisiana	Describes the location of items/areas in the classroom and places in home and community.	Concepts Describe Prepositions
	Kansas	Questions why and/or how people are similar or different.	Ask questions Compare/contrast
	District of Columbia	Demonstrates a basic understanding of sequence of events and time periods (e.g., using terms such as time of day, yesterday, today, and tomorrow).	Concepts Sequence
	Tennessee	Begins to categorize time intervals. Uses word "today," or "day" and "night" to talk about time of day, sometimes uses the wrong term.	Concepts Categorize
	Louisiana	Uses words to describe events or activities that happened at an earlier time (e.g., "after we had snack" or "last night").	Describe Concepts Sequence
	Louisiana	Tells why rules are important.	Cause/effect
	District of Columbia	Demonstrates beginning understanding of commerce through exploring the roles of buying and selling in play.	Concepts Cause/effect
Cognition	Georgia	Intentionally carries out an action with an understanding of the effect it will cause.	Cause/effect
	Rhode Island	Communicates with some detail about events that happened in the past.	Past tense Sequence Supporting details

3 Year Olds *continued*

Area	State	Early Learning Standard	Speech and Language Skills
Cognition	Rhode Island	With support, retells or reenacts familiar stories, including such details as characters, phrases, and events.	Retell Narrative elements
	Georgia	Uses clues and sequence of events to infer and predict what will happen next.	Sequence Infer/draw conclusion Predict
	North Carolina	Recognizes whether a picture of an object is the same as or different from something they have seen before.	Compare/contrast
	Carolina	Describes or acts out a memory of a situation or action, with adult support.	Describe
	North Carolina	Asks questions about why things happen and tries to understand cause and effect.	Ask questions Cause/effect
	Rhode Island	Solves simple problems without trying every possibility (e.g., putting big blocks at the base of a tower and smaller blocks on top to make a tower that doesn't topple).	Problem solve
Approaches to Learning	Louisiana	Asks adults for help on tasks, if needed.	Request help, information, clarification
	Louisiana	Asks more complex questions for clarification and to seek meaningful information.	Request help, information, clarification
	North Carolina	Uses language to begin and carry on play with others.	Pragmatics
	North Carolina	Purposefully uses a variety of strategies to solve different types of problems.	Problem solve

3 Year Olds *continued*

Area	State	Early Learning Standard	Speech and Language Skills
Social-Emotional	Georgia	Uses a combination of words, phrases, and actions to communicate needs, ideas, opinions, and preferences.	Vocabulary Syntax/morphology Pragmatics
	Kansas	Describes situations which can elicit various emotions (e.g., tells a story that is supposed to make a listener sad).	Describe
	North Carolina	Describes self (characteristics that can be seen, things they can do, things they like, possessions).	Describe Identify own emotions
	Rhode Island	Suggests solutions to conflicts, with adult guidance and assistance.	Problem solve
	Georgia	With adult guidance, uses verbal and non-verbal expressions to demonstrate a larger range of emotions such as frustration, jealousy, and enthusiasm.	Identify own emotions Nonverbal cues
	North Carolina	Demonstrates social skills when interacting with other children (turn taking, conflict resolution, sharing).	Pragmatics
	Rhode Island	Initiates play and conversations with other children.	Initiating conversation
	North Carolina	Expresses a range of emotions (happiness, sadness, fear, anger, disgust, tenderness, hostility, shame, guilt, satisfaction, and love) with their face, body, vocal sounds, and words.	Identify own emotions
	North Carolina	Communicates concern for others (share a toy with someone who doesn't have one, ask, "Are you OK?").	Taking perspective of others
	Rhode Island	Expresses how another child or storybook character might feel.	Taking perspective of others

4 YEAR OLDS

Area	State	Early Learning Standard	Speech and Language Skills
Communication and Literacy	Georgia	Listens to and follows multistep directions.	Concepts Sequence
	Kansas	Demonstrates an understanding of some frequently occurring verbs and adjectives by relating them to their opposites (e.g., up, down, stop, go, in, out).	Verbs Adjectives Antonyms
	Kansas	Distinguishes among some verbs describing the same general action (e.g., walk, march, strut, prance) by acting out the meanings.	Verbs Synonyms
	Louisiana	Uses new vocabulary acquired through conversations, activities, or listening to texts read aloud.	Vocabulary
	Tennessee	Recognizes that some words have more than one meaning as used in a conversation or as found in a book (i.e., bank, a place to keep money, and bank the edge of a river).	Multiple meaning words
	Tennessee	With guidance and support, identifies the role of the author and the illustrator.	Nouns Verbs
	Tennessee	Sorts familiar objects into categories and identifies the "common" factor of the group (e.g. identifies reason {common factor} for grouping objects; categorizes animals by those who fly or walk; groups cars by color or number of doors).	Sort Categorize
	Kansas	Uses some basic spatial (e.g., front/back, top/bottom) and temporal (e.g., first/last, before/after) concepts to describe familiar people, places, things, and events.	Concepts Describe
	Kansas	Uses the many frequently occurring prepositions (e.g., to, from, in, out, on, off, for, of, by, with).	Concepts Prepositions

4 Year Olds *continued*

Area	State	Early Learning Standard	Speech and Language Skills
Communication and Literacy	District of Columbia	Determines the meanings of unknown words/ concepts using the context of conversations, pictures or concrete objects.	Meaning from context
	Head Start	With increasing independence, matches the tone and volume of expression to the content and social situation, such as by using a whisper to tell a secret.	Nonverbal cues
	Head Start	Uses verbal and non-verbal signals appropriately to acknowledge the comments or questions of others.	Responding Nonverbal cues
	Georgia	Describes activities, experiences, and stories with more detail.	Describe
	Georgia	Develops an alternate ending for a story.	Sequence Infer/draw conclusions
	Kansas	Understands and uses most question words (i.e., interrogatives) (e.g., who, what, where, when, why, how).	Ask questions Answer questions
	Kansas	With prompting and support answers "why" questions based on information presented in the text.	Answer questions
	Tennessee	With modeling and guidance, asks and answers questions in order to seek help, get information, or clarify something which is not understood.	Ask questions Answer questions Request help, information, clarification
	Louisiana	With prompting and support, describes what person, place, thing, or idea in the text an illustration depicts.	Describe
	Kansas	With prompting and support, identifies characters, settings, and major events in a story.	Narrative elements

4 Year Olds *continued*

Area	State	Early Learning Standard	Speech and Language Skills
Communication and Literacy	Kansas	With prompting and support, asks and answers questions about key details in a text.	Ask questions Answer questions Important versus unimportant details
	Head Start	Answers questions about details of a story with increasingly specific information, such as when asked, "Who was Mary?" responds, "She was the girl who was riding the horse and then got hurt."	Answer questions
	Kansas	With prompting and support, retells key details of a text.	Important versus unimportant details Retell
	Kansas	With prompting and support, begins to compare and contrast the adventures and experiences of characters in familiar stories.	Compare/contrast
	Kansas	With prompting and support, describes the connection between two events or pieces of information in a text.	Describe Compare/contrast
	Kansas	With prompting and support, identifies a similarity and difference between two texts on the same topic (e.g., in illustrations, descriptions, or procedures).	Compare/contrast
	Louisiana	With prompting and support, discusses basic similarities and differences in print read aloud, including characters, settings, events, and ideas.	Compare/contrast Narrative elements
	Louisiana	Uses a combination of drawing, dictating, and/or writing in response to a text read aloud, or to tell a story about a life experience or event.	Describe Retell
	Rhode Island	Retells a familiar story in the proper sequence, including major events and cause-and-effect relationships.	Retell Sequence Cause/effect Narrative elements Important versus unimportant details

4 Year Olds *continued*

Area	State	Early Learning Standard	Speech and Language Skills
Communication and Literacy	Rhode Island	Engages in higher-order thinking during shared reading experiences, such as making predictions and inferences, determining cause-and-effect relationships, and summarizing stories.	Predict Infer/draw conclusions Cause/effect Summarize
	Head Start	Produces the beginning sound in a spoken word, such as "Dog begins with /d/."	Concepts
	Kansas	With prompting and support, blends and segments initial sounds (i.e., onset) and ending sounds (i.e., rime) of single syllable words (e.g., /d/+/og/ = dog).	Concepts
	Kansas	States the initial sound (phoneme) in consonant-vowel-consonant (CVC) words (e.g., cat starts with /c/).	Concepts
	Head Start	Shows understanding of a variety of sentence types, such as multiclause, cause-effect, sequential order, or if-then.	Sequence Cause/effect Syntax/morphology
	North Carolina	Shows understanding of increasingly complex sentences.	Syntax/morphology
	Head Start	Shows an understanding of talk related to the past or future.	Past tense Future tense
	Rhode Island	Uses increasingly complex, longer sentences, including sentences that combine two or three phrases.	Syntax/morphology

4 Year Olds *continued*

Area	State	Early Learning Standard	Speech and Language Skills
Communication and Literacy	Rhode Island	Uses more complex grammar and parts of speech, including prepositions, regular and irregular plural forms of nouns, correct subject-verb agreement, pronouns, possessives, and regular and irregular past tense verbs.	Nouns Verbs Prepositions Past tense Plurals Pronouns Possessives Present tense Sentence construction
	Rhode Island	Communicates clearly enough to be understood by unfamiliar listeners, with few pronunciation errors.	Articulation/ phonological processes
	Head Start	Uses language, spoken or sign, to clarify a word or statement when misunderstood.	Conversational repairs
	North Carolina	Uses language and nonverbal cues to communicate thoughts, beliefs, feelings, and intentions.	Pragmatics
	Tennessee	Observes and uses appropriate ways of interacting in a group (e.g., taking turns in talking, actively listening to peers, waiting to speak until another person is finished talking, asking questions and waiting for an answer).	Pragmatics
	Rhode Island	Engages, with support and modeling, in conversations of at least five turns, with each exchange relating to and building upon what was said previously.	Responding Initiating conversation Topic maintenance
Math	Kansas	Counts to answer "how many?" questions about as many as 10 things arranged in a line, a rectangular array or a circle or as many as five things in a scattered configuration.	Answer questions

4 Year Olds *continued*

Area	State	Early Learning Standard	Speech and Language Skills
Math	Tennessee	Uses comparative language, such as more/less than or equal to, to compare and describe collections of objects by matching.	Comparatives/superlatives Compare/contrast Describe
	Louisiana	Uses and understands positions of objects, self and other people in space, including in/on, over/under, up/down, inside/outside, beside/between, and in front/behind.	Concepts Prepositions
	Georgia	Uses appropriate directional language to indicate where things are in their environment — positions, distances, order (behind, in front of, next to, left, right, over, under).	Concepts Prepositions
	Tennessee	Explores the concept of measurement to compare the attributes of two or more concrete objects and uses words to define attributes of the objects (i.e. heavier/lighter, longer/shorter, covers more/covers less, holds more/holds less).	Adjectives Comparatives/superlatives Compare/contrast
	North Carolina	Shows they understand that putting two groups of objects together will make a bigger group and that a group of objects can be taken apart into smaller groups.	Comparatives/superlatives
	North Carolina	Shows understanding of first, next, and last during play and daily activities (answer questions about who is first and last to slide down the slide; say, "The engine is first, and the caboose is last" when making a train).	Answer questions Concepts Sequence
	Georgia	Tells numbers that come before and after a given number up to 10.	Sequence
	Georgia	Matches two equal sets using one-to-one correspondence and understands they are the same.	Match Compare/contrast

4 Year Olds *continued*

Area	State	Early Learning Standard	Speech and Language Skills
Math	Kansas	Collects data by categories to answer simple questions.	Answer questions Categorize
	Louisiana	Sorts objects by more than one attribute (e.g., red circles or blue triangles) and explains the criteria used to sort objects.	Sort Categorize Adjectives
	Louisiana	Identifies and names simple measurement tools and describes what they are used for (e.g., ruler measures length, scale measures weight).	Nouns Describe
	Louisiana	Identifies and names at least the four basic shapes (rectangles, squares, circles, and triangles) when presented using different sizes and in different orientations.	Nouns
	Louisiana	Describes and names attributes of four basic shapes (e.g., a square has four equal sides, a circle is round).	Concepts Describe
	Head Start	Identifies and uses numbers related to order or position from first to tenth.	Concepts Sequence
Science	Louisiana	Uses all five senses to observe, collect information, describe observations, classify based on observations, and form conclusions about what is observed.	Describe Categorize Infer/draw conclusions
	Tennessee	Describes and categorizes objects based on their observable properties.	Describe Categorize
	Kansas	Describes and compares the effects of common forces (e.g., pushes and pulls) on objects and the impact of gravity, magnetism and mechanical forces (e.g., ramps, gears, pendulums, and other simple machines).	Describe Compare/contrast Cause/effect
	Kansas	Asks/answers questions about objects, organisms, and events in their environments.	Ask questions Answer questions

4 Year Olds *continued*

Area	State	Early Learning Standard	Speech and Language Skills
Science	Louisiana	Uses basic vocabulary to name and describe plants and living creatures.	Vocabulary Describe
	Georgia	Identifies and describes the functions of many body parts.	Nouns Verbs Adjectives Describe
	North Carolina	Compares objects, materials, and phenomena by observing and describing their physical characteristics.	Describe Compare/contrast
	Rhode Island	Describes the characteristics that define living things.	Adjectives Describe
	Rhode Island	Observes the similarities, differences, and categories of plants and animals.	Categorize Compare/contrast
	Louisiana	Uses basic vocabulary to describe similarities and differences between living creatures and plants.	Vocabulary Compare/contrast
	Rhode Island	Describes changes that occur in the natural environment over time.	Concepts Describe Sequence
	Kansas	Understands and is able to explain why plants and animals need air, food, and water.	Answer questions
	Louisiana	Shows an understanding of cause and effect relationships and uses this understanding to predict what will happen as a result of an action and to solve simple problems.	Cause/effect Predict Problem solve
	Louisiana	Uses prior knowledge and experiences to generate questions, hypothesize, predict, and draw conclusions about living creatures, objects, materials and changes observed in the environment.	Ask questions Predict Infer/draw conclusions

4 Year Olds *continued*

Area	State	Early Learning Standard	Speech and Language Skills
Science	Louisiana	With prompting and support, uses scientific vocabulary words to describe steps in the scientific process (e.g., "observation," "experiment," "hypothesis," "conclusion").	Vocabulary Describe Sequence
	Kansas	Demonstrates an understanding that different weather conditions require different clothing/accessories (e.g., boots, mittens, raincoat).	Vocabulary Cause/effect
	Head Start	Asks questions that can be answered through an investigation, such as, "What do plants need to grow?" or "What countries do the children in our class come from?"	Ask questions
	Head Start	Articulates steps to be taken and lists materials needed for an investigation or experiment.	Vocabulary Sequence
	Head Start	Gathers information about a question by looking at books or discussing prior knowledge and observations.	Answer questions
	Head Start	Analyzes and interprets data and summarizes results of investigation.	Summarize Infer/draw conclusions
	Head Start	Draws conclusions, constructs explanations, and verbalizes cause and effect relationships.	Describe Cause/effect Infer/draw conclusions
	Head Start	With adult support, compares results to initial prediction and offers evidence as to why they do or do not work.	Compare/contrast Predict Infer/draw conclusions
	Head Start	Generates new testable questions based on results.	Ask questions
	Louisiana	Compares and contrasts seasonal changes where they live.	Compare/contrast

4 Year Olds *continued*

Area	State	Early Learning Standard	Speech and Language Skills
Science	Louisiana	Describes the current weather and how weather conditions can change from day to day.	Adjectives Describe
	Louisiana	Describes major features of the earth and sky, and how they change from night to day.	Describe
	District of Columbia	Begins to distinguish evidence from opinion.	Fact/opinion
Social Studies	Louisiana	Identifies workers and their roles as citizens within the community.	Vocabulary
	Tennessee	Develops an understanding of how people and things change over time.	Concepts Sequence
	District of Columbia	Demonstrates a beginning understanding of past, present and future as it relates to one's self, family, and community.	Concepts Sequence Past tense Present tense Future tense
	Kansas	Identifies and correctly uses terms related to location, direction, and distance (e.g., up/down, here/there).	Concepts Prepositions
	Kansas	Matches objects to usual locations and identifies features of familiar places (e.g., tree in a park, bed in a bedroom).	Vocabulary Match Categorize
	Kansas	Describes some of the holidays, foods, and special events related to his/her own culture or acts them out in dramatic play.	Vocabulary Describe
	Rhode Island	Makes comparisons about similarities and differences among people and uses themselves as a reference (e.g., saying, "That boy is bigger than me!").	Comparatives/superlatives Compare/contrast
	Rhode Island	Uses and understands concepts of "before" and "after."	Concepts Sequence

4 Year Olds *continued*

Area	State	Early Learning Standard	Speech and Language Skills
Social Studies	Rhode Island	Uses such terms as "today," "tomorrow," and "next time" with some accuracy.	Concepts Sequence
	Kansas	Demonstrates an understanding that money can be exchanged for goods and services.	Cause/effect
Cognition	North Carolina	Organizes and uses information through matching, grouping, and sequencing.	Match Categorize Sequence
	North Carolina	Describes past events in an organized way, including details or personal reactions.	Concepts Describe Sequence Supporting details
	Rhode Island	Retells a familiar story in the proper sequence, including such details as characters, phrases, and events.	Retell Sequence Narrative elements Supporting details
	Rhode Island	Remembers more and more minute details from a story and is able to answer questions accurately (e.g., "How did the peddler feel when the monkeys didn't give him back his caps?").	Answer questions Important versus unimportant details
	Georgia	Recognizes cause-and-effect relationships.	Cause/effect
	Georgia	Explains why simple events occur using reasoning skills (why).	Cause/effect Infer/draw conclusions
	Georgia	Draws conclusions based on facts and evidence.	Infer/draw conclusions
	Georgia	Makes, checks and verifies predictions.	Predict
	District of Columbia	Generates or seeks out multiple solutions to a problem.	Problem solve

4 Year Olds *continued*

Area	State	Early Learning Standard	Speech and Language Skills
Cognition	North Carolina	Expresses understanding that others may have different thoughts, beliefs, or feelings than their own ("I like ketchup and you don't.").	Taking perspective of others
	Tennessee	Seeks additional clarity to further own knowledge (e.g., asks what, how, why, when, where, and/or what if).	Ask questions
Approaches to Learning	Louisiana	Makes specific request for help from both peers and adults as needed.	Request help, information, clarification
	North Carolina	Seeks assistance and/or information when needed to complete a task.	Request help, information, clarification
	Kansas	Identifies a problem, demonstrates flexibility in solving it and changes plans if a better solution is proposed.	Problem Solve
	North Carolina	Describes the steps they will use to solve a problem.	Describe Sequence Problem solve
	Georgia	Effectively uses words, sentences and actions to communicate needs, ideas, opinions, and preferences.	Vocabulary Syntax/ morphology Pragmatics
Social-Emotional	Kansas	Describes characteristics of self and others.	Describe
	North Carolina	Makes requests clearly and effectively most of the time.	Request for object or action
	Kansas	Recognizes and respects similarities and differences between self and others (e.g., gender, race, special needs, cultures, languages, family structures).	Compare/contrast
	Louisiana	Demonstrates understanding of how one's words and actions affect others.	Cause/effect

4 Year Olds *continued*

Area	State	Early Learning Standard	Speech and Language Skills
Social-Emotional	North Carolina	Uses a variety of strategies to solve problems and conflicts with increasing independence.	Problem solve
	Kansas	Participates in conversational turn taking by listening and responding to what was said.	Responding Topic maintenance
	Rhode Island	Participates in longer and more reciprocal interactions (when interacting with familiar adults in role play, games, or structured activities) and takes greater initiative in social interaction (including turn-taking).	Pragmatics
	North Carolina	Expresses a range of emotions (happiness, sadness, fear, anger, disgust, tenderness, hostility, shame, guilt, satisfaction, and love) with their face, body, vocal sounds, and words.	Vocabulary Nonverbal cues Identify own emotions
	Rhode Island	Can predict the causes of other children's emotions (e.g., "she is sad because . . . ").	Predict Cause/effect Taking perspective of others

2

Common Core State Standards (CCSS)

The Common Core State Standards (CCSS) that have been selected in this chapter require a strong foundation of speech-language skills. The standards are organized by grade level and the following Common Core areas (NGA Center & CCSSO, 2010):

- RL—Reading: Literature

- RI—Reading: Informational Text

- RF—Reading: Foundational Skills

- W—Writing

- SL—Speaking & Listening

- L—Language

- CC—Math: Counting & Cardinality

- OA—Math: Operations & Algebraic Thinking

- NBT—Math: Number & Operations in Base Ten

- NF—Math: Number & Operations-Fractions

- MD—Measurement & Data

- G—Math: Geometry

- RP—Math: Ratios & Proportional Relationships

- NS—Math: The Number System

- EE—Math: Expressions & Equations

- F—Math: Functions

- SP—Math: Statistics & Probability

- RH—Reading Standards for Literacy in History/Social Studies

- RST—Reading Standards for Literacy in Science & Technical Subjects

Each standard includes the area, number of the standard as indicated in the CCSS and the specific prerequisite speech and language skill(s). The speech-language pathologist (SLP) will use this chapter to help identify the *Prerequisite Skills* a student is lacking. There are times when just pragmatics or syntax and morphology are indicated for the prerequisite speech-language skills. When this happens, it is referring to *all* pragmatic skills or *all* syntax and morphology skills. The next step is to proceed to Chapter 3 to locate the *Prerequisite Skills* and *Steps to Mastery*.

For those SLPs whose state or school system has not adopted the Common Core State Standards, this chapter can be compared to their adopted curriculum standards. This can assist SLPs in identifying prerequisite skills in those standards.

KINDERGARTEN

Area	#	Common Core State Standard	Speech & Language Skills
RL RI	1	With prompting and support, ask and answer questions about key details in a text.	Ask questions Answer questions
RL	2	With prompting and support, retell familiar stories, including key details.	Retell Important versus unimportant details
RL	3	With prompting and support, identify characters, settings, and major events in a story.	Narrative elements
RL	4	Ask and answer questions about unknown words in a text.	Ask questions Answer questions Meaning from context
RL	6	With prompting and support, name the author and illustrator of a story and define the role of each in telling the story.	Describe
RL	9	With prompting and support, compare and contrast the adventures and experiences of characters in familiar stories.	Compare/contrast
RI	2	With prompting and support, identify the main topic and retell key details of a text.	Main idea Retell Important versus unimportant details
RI	3	With prompting and support, describe the connection between two individuals, events, ideas, or pieces of information in a text.	Compare/contrast
RI	4	With prompting and support, ask and answer questions about unknown words in a text.	Ask questions Answer questions Meaning from context

Kindergarten *continued*

Area	#	Common Core State Standard	Speech & Language Skills
RI	6	Name the author and illustrator of a text and define the role of each in presenting the ideas or information in a text.	Describe
RI	7	With prompting and support, describe the relationship between illustrations and the text in which they appear.	Describe Compare/contrast
RI	8	With prompting and support, identify the reasons an author gives to support points in a text.	Supporting details
RI	9	With prompting and support, identify basic similarities in and differences between two texts on the same topic.	Compare/contrast
RF	1	Demonstrate understanding of the organization and basic features of print. a. Follow words from left to right, top to bottom, and page by page.	Concepts
W	1	Use a combination of drawing, dictating, and writing to compose opinion pieces in which they tell a reader the topic or the name of the book they are writing about and state an opinion or preference about the topic or book.	Fact/opinion Main idea
W	2	Use a combination of drawing, dictating, and writing to compose informative/explanatory texts in which they name what they are writing about and supply some information about the topic.	Main idea Supporting details
W	3	Use a combination of drawing, dictating, and writing to narrate a single event or several loosely linked events, tell about the events in the order in which they occurred, and provide a reaction to what happened.	Describe Sequence
W	5	With guidance and support from adults, respond to questions and suggestions from peers and add details to strengthen writing as needed.	Answer questions
W	6	With guidance and support from adults, explore a variety of digital tools to produce and publish writing, including in collaboration with peers.	Pragmatics

Kindergarten *continued*

Area	#	Common Core State Standard	Speech & Language Skills
W	7	Participate in shared research and writing projects.	Pragmatics
SL	1	Participate in collaborative conversations with diverse partners about *kindergarten topics and texts* with peers and adults in small and larger groups. a. Follow agreed-upon rules for discussions. b. Continue a conversation through multiple exchanges.	Pragmatics
SL	2	Confirm understanding of a text read aloud or information presented orally or through other media by asking and answering questions about key details and requesting clarification if something is not understood.	Ask questions Answer questions Request help, information, clarification
SL	3	Ask and answer questions in order to seek help, get information, or clarify something that is not understood.	Ask questions Answer questions Request help, information, clarification
SL	4	Describe familiar people, places, things, and events and, with prompting and support, provide additional detail.	Describe
SL	6	Speak audibly and express thoughts, feelings, and ideas clearly.	Pragmatics
L	1	Demonstrate command of the conventions of standard English grammar and usage when writing or speaking. b. Use frequently occurring nouns and verbs. c. Form regular plural nouns orally by adding /s/ or /es/. d. Understand and use question words (interrogatives). e. Use the most frequently occurring prepositions. f. Produce and expand complete sentences in shared language activities.	Nouns Verbs Plurals Ask questions Answer questions Concepts Sentence construction

Kindergarten *continued*

Area	#	Common Core State Standard	Speech & Language Skills
L	4	Determine or clarify the meaning of unknown and multiple-meaning words and phrases based on *kindergarten reading and content*. a. Identify new meaning for familiar words and apply them accurately. b. Use the most frequently occurring inflections and affixes as a clue to the meaning of an unknown word.	Describe Meaning from context Word parts Multiple meaning words
L	5	With guidance and support from adults, explore word relationships and nuances in word meanings. a. Sort common objects into categories to gain a sense of the concepts the categories represent. b. Demonstrate understanding of frequently occurring verbs and adjectives by relating them to their opposites (antonyms). c. Identify real-life connections between words and their use. d. Distinguish shades of meaning among verbs describing the same general action by acting out the meanings.	Sort Describe Categorize Verbs Adjectives
L	6	Use words and phrases acquired through conversations, reading and being read to, and responding to texts.	Vocabulary
CC	B5	Count to answer "how many?" questions about as many as 20 things arranged in a line, a rectangular array, or a circle, or as many as 10 things in a scattered configuration; given a number from 1 to 20, count out that many objects.	Answer questions Concepts
CC	C7	Compare two numbers between 1 and 10 presented as written numerals.	Compare/contrast
OA	A3	Decompose numbers less than or equal to 10 into pairs in more than one way.	Concepts

Kindergarten *continued*

Area	#	Common Core State Standard	Speech & Language Skills
MD	A1	Describe measurable attributes of objects, such as length or weight. Describe several measurable attributes of a single object.	Adjectives Describe
MD	A2	Directly compare two objects with a measurable attribute in common, to see which object has "more of"/"less of" the attribute, and describe the difference.	Concepts Describe Compare/contrast
MD	B3	Classify objects into given categories; count the numbers of objects in each category and sort the categories by count.	Sort Categorize
G	A1	Describe objects in the environment using names of shapes, and describe the relative positions of these objects using terms such as above, below, beside, in front of, behind, and next to.	Concepts Describe
G	A2	Correctly name shapes regardless of their orientations or overall size.	Nouns Adjectives
G	B4	Analyze and compare two- and three-dimensional shapes, in different sizes and orientations, using informal language to describe their similarities, differences, parts and other attributes.	Compare/contrast Describe Adjectives

1ST GRADE

Area	#	Common Core State Standard	Speech & Language Skills
RL RI	1	Ask and answer questions about key details in a text.	Ask questions Answer questions
RL	2	Retell stories, including key details, and demonstrate understanding of their central message or lesson.	Main idea Retell Important versus unimportant details
RL	3	Describe characters, settings, and major events in a story, using key details.	Describe Narrative elements Important versus unimportant details
RL	5	Explain major differences between books that tell stories and books that give information, drawing on a wide reading of a range of text types.	Compare/contrast
RL	9	Compare and contrast the adventures and experiences of characters in stories.	Compare/contrast
RI	2	Identify the main topic and retell key details of a text.	Main idea Retell Important versus unimportant details
RI	3	Describe the connection between two individuals, events, ideas, or pieces of information in a text.	Compare/contrast
RI	4	Ask and answer questions to help determine or clarify the meaning of words and phrases in a text.	Ask questions Answer questions Meaning from context
RI	7	Use the illustrations and details in a text to describe its key ideas.	Describe Important versus unimportant details

1st Grade *continued*

Area	#	Common Core State Standard	Speech & Language Skills
RI	8	Identify the reasons an author gives to support points in a text.	Supporting details
RI	9	Identify basic similarities in and differences between two texts on the same topic.	Compare/contrast
RF	2	Demonstrate understanding of spoken words, syllables, and sounds (phonemes). c. Isolate and pronounce initial, medial vowel, and final sounds (phonemes) in spoken single-syllable words.	Articulation/ phonological processes
W	1	Write opinion pieces in which they introduce the topic or name the book they are writing about, state an opinion, supply a reason for the opinion, and provide some sense of closure.	Fact/opinion Main idea Supporting details
W	2	Write informative/explanatory texts in which they name a topic, supply some facts about the topic, and provide some sense of closure.	Main idea Supporting details
W	3	Write narratives in which they recount two or more appropriately sequenced events, include some details regarding what happened, use temporal words to signal event order, and provide some sense of closure.	Concepts Sequence Supporting details
W	5	With guidance and support from adults, focus on a topic, respond to questions and suggestions from peers, and add details to strengthen writing as needed.	Main idea Answer questions Supporting details
W	6	With guidance and support from adults, use a variety of digital tools to produce and publish writing, including in collaboration with peers.	Pragmatics
W	7	Participate in shared research and writing projects.	Pragmatics
W	8	With guidance and support from adults, recall information from experiences or gather information from provided sources to answer a question.	Answer questions

1st Grade *continued*

Area	#	Common Core State Standard	Speech & Language Skills
SL	1	Participate in collaborative conversations with diverse partners about *grade 1 topics and texts* with peers and adults in small and larger groups. a. Follow agreed-upon rules for discussions. b. Build on others' talk in conversations by responding to the comments of others through multiple exchanges. c. Ask questions to clear up any confusion about the topics and texts under discussion.	Pragmatics Ask questions
SL	2	Ask and answer questions about key details in a text read aloud or information presented orally or through other media.	Ask questions Answer questions
SL	3	Ask and answer questions about what a speaker says in order to gather additional information or clarify something that is not understood.	Ask questions Answer questions Request help, information, clarification
SL	4	Describe people, places, things, and events with relevant details, expressing ideas and feelings clearly.	Describe
SL	6	Produce complete sentences when appropriate to task and situation.	Sentence construction
L	1	Demonstrate command of the conventions of standard English grammar and usage when writing or speaking. b. Use common, proper, and possessive nouns. c. Use singular and plural nouns with matching verbs in basic sentences. d. Use personal, possessive, and indefinite pronouns. e. Use verbs to convey a sense of past, present, and future. f. Use frequently occurring adjectives. g. Use frequently occurring conjunctions. i. Use frequently occurring prepositions. j. Produce and expand complete simple and compound declarative, interrogative, imperative, and exclamatory sentences in response to prompts.	Possessives Nouns Plurals Pronouns Verbs Past tense Present tense Future tense Adjectives Conjunctions Sentence construction

1st Grade *continued*

Area	#	Common Core State Standard	Speech & Language Skills
L	4	Determine or clarify the meaning of unknown and multiple-meaning words and phrases based on *grade 1 reading and content*, choosing flexibly from an array of strategies. a. Use sentence-level context as a clue to the meaning of a word or phrase. b. Use frequently occurring affixes as a clue to the meaning of a word. c. Identify frequently occurring root words and their inflectional forms.	Meaning from context Word parts
L	5	With guidance and support from adults, demonstrate understanding of word relationships and nuances in word meaning. a. Sort words into categories to gain a sense of the concepts the categories represent. b. Define words by category and by one or more key attributes. c. Identify real-life connections between words and their use. d. Distinguish shades of meaning among verbs differing in manner and adjectives differing in intensity by defining or choosing them or by acting out the meanings.	Sort Describe Compare/contrast Categorize Verbs Adjectives
L	6	Use words and phrases acquired through conversations, reading and being read to, and responding to texts, including using frequently occurring conjunctions to signal simple relationships.	Vocabulary Conjunctions
OA	A1	Use addition and subtraction within 20 to solve word problems involving situations of adding to, taking from, putting together, taking apart, and comparing, with unknowns in all positions.	Concepts Compare/contrast
OA	A2	Solve word problems that call for addition of three whole numbers whose sum is less than or equal to 20.	Concepts

1st Grade *continued*

Area	#	Common Core State Standard	Speech & Language Skills
OA	C6	Add and subtract within 20, demonstrating fluency for addition and subtraction within 10. Use strategies such as counting on; making ten; decomposing a number leading to a ten; using the relationship between addition and subtraction; and creating equivalent but easier or known sums.	Compare/contrast
OA	D7	Understand the meaning of the equal sign, and determine if equations involving addition and subtraction are true or false.	Concepts
NBT	B3	Compare two two-digit numbers based on meanings of the tens and ones digits, recording the results of comparisons with the symbols >, =, and <.	Compare/contrast
NBT	C4	Add within 100, including adding a two-digit number and a one-digit number, and adding a two-digit number and a multiple of 10, using concrete models or drawings and strategies based on place value, properties of operations, and/or the relationship between addition and subtraction; relate the strategy to a written method and explain the reasoning used. Understand that in adding two-digit numbers, one adds tens and tens, ones and ones; and sometimes it is necessary to compose a ten.	Compare/contrast Infer/draw conclusions
NBT	C5	Given a two-digit number, mentally find 10 more or 10 less than the number, without having to count; explain the reasoning used.	Concepts Infer/draw conclusions
NBT	C6	Subtract multiples of 10 in the range 10 to 90 from multiples of 10 in the range 10 to 90 (positive or zero differences), using concrete models or drawings and strategies based on place value, properties of operations, and/or the relationship between addition and subtraction; relate the strategy to a written method and explain the reasoning used.	Compare/contrast Infer/draw conclusions
MD	A1	Order three objects by length; compare the lengths of two objects indirectly by using a third object.	Compare/contrast

1st Grade *continued*

Area	#	Common Core State Standard	Speech & Language Skills
MD	C4	Organize, represent, and interpret data with up to three categories; ask and answer questions about the total number of data points, how many in each category, and how many more or less are in one category than in another.	Concepts Categorize Ask questions Answer questions
G	A1	Distinguish between defining attributes versus non-defining attributes; build and draw shapes to possess defining attributes.	Adjectives
G	A3	Partition circles and rectangles into two and four equal shares, describe the shares using the words halves, fourths, and quarters, and use the phrases half of, fourth of, and quarter of. Describe the whole as two of, or four of the shares. Understand for these examples that decomposing into more equal shares creates smaller shares.	Concepts Describe

2ND GRADE

Area	#	Common Core State Standard	Speech & Language Skills
RL RI	1	Ask and answer such questions as who, what, where, when, why, and how to demonstrate understanding of key details in a text.	Ask questions Answer questions
RL	2	Recount stories, including fables and folktales from diverse cultures, and determine their central message, lesson, or moral.	Retell Main idea
RL	3	Describe how characters in a story respond to major events and challenges.	Describe
RL	4	Describe how words and phrases supply rhythm and meaning in a story, poem, or song.	Describe
RL	5	Describe the overall structure of a story, including describing how the beginning introduces the story and the ending concludes the action.	Describe Sequence
RL	6	Acknowledge differences in the points of view of characters, including by speaking in a different voice for each character when reading dialogue aloud.	Compare/contrast Taking perspective of others
RL	9	Compare and contrast two or more versions of the same story by different authors or from different cultures.	Compare/contrast
RI	2	Identify the main topic of a multiparagraph text as well as the focus of specific paragraphs within the text.	Main idea
RI	3	Describe the connection between a series of historical events, scientific ideas or concepts, or steps in technical procedures in a text.	Compare/contrast
RI	4	Determine the meaning of words and phrases in a text relevant to a *grade 2 topic or subject area*.	Meaning from context
RI	6	Identify the main purpose of a text, including what the author wants to answer, explain, or describe.	Main idea

2nd Grade *continued*

Area	#	Common Core State Standard	Speech & Language Skills
RI	8	Describe how reasons support specific points the author makes in a text.	Describe Supporting details
RI	9	Compare and contrast the most important points presented by two texts on the same topic.	Compare/contrast Important versus unimportant details
W	1	Write opinion pieces in which they introduce the topic or book they are writing about, state an opinion, supply reasons that support the opinion, use linking words to connect opinion and reasons, and provide a concluding statement or section.	Main idea Fact/opinion Supporting details Conjunctions
W	2	Write informative/explanatory texts in which they introduce a topic, use facts and definitions to develop points, and provide a concluding statement or section.	Main idea Supporting details Sequence
W	3	Write narratives in which they recount a well-elaborated event or short sequence of events, include details to describe actions, thoughts, and feelings, use temporal words to signal event order, and provide a sense of closure.	Concepts Sequence Retell Supporting details
W	5	With guidance and support from adults and peers, focus on a topic and strengthen writing as needed by revising and editing.	Main idea
W	6	With guidance and support from adults, use a variety of digital tools to produce and publish writing, including in collaboration with peers.	Pragmatics
W	7	Participate in shared research and writing projects.	Pragmatics
W	8	Recall information from experiences or gather information from provided sources to answer a question.	Answer questions

2nd Grade *continued*

Area	#	Common Core State Standard	Speech & Language Skills
SL	1	Participate in collaborative conversations with diverse partners about grade 2 topics and texts with peers and adults in small and large groups. a. Follow agreed-upon rules for discussions. b. Build on others' talk in conversation by linking their comments to the remarks of others. c. Ask for clarification and further explanation as needed about the topics and texts under discussion.	Pragmatics Ask questions
SL	2	Recount or describe key ideas or details from a text read aloud or information presented orally or through other media.	Retell Describe Important versus unimportant details
SL	3	Ask and answer questions about what a speaker says in order to clarify comprehension, gather additional information, or deepen understanding of a topic or issue.	Ask questions Answer questions Request help, information, clarification
SL	4	Tell a story or recount an experience with appropriate key facts and relevant, descriptive details, speaking audibly in coherent sentences.	Retell Main idea Supporting details Syntax & morphology
SL	6	Produce complete sentences when appropriate to task and situation in order to provide requested detail or clarification.	Sentence construction Answer questions

2nd Grade *continued*

Area	#	Common Core State Standard	Speech & Language Skills
L	1	Demonstrate command of the conventions of standard English grammar and usage when writing or speaking. a. Use collective nouns. b. Form and use frequently occurring irregular plural nouns. c. Use reflexive pronouns. d. Form and use the past tense of frequently occurring irregular verbs. e. Use adjectives and adverbs, and choose between them depending on what is to be modified. f. Produce, expand, and rearrange complete simple and compound sentences.	Nouns Plurals Pronouns Past tense Adjectives Adverbs Sentence construction
L	3	Use knowledge of language and its conventions when writing, speaking, reading, or listening.	Syntax/morphology
L	4	Determine or clarify the meaning of unknown and multiple-meaning words and phrases based on *grade 2 reading and content*, choosing flexibly from an array of strategies. a. Use sentence-level context as a clue to the meaning of a word or phrase. b. Determine the meaning of the new word formed when a known prefix is added to a known word. c. Use a known root word as a clue to the meaning of an unknown word with the same root. d. Use knowledge of the meaning of individual words to predict the meaning of compound words. e. Use glossaries and beginning dictionaries, both print and digital, to determine or clarify the meaning of words and phrases.	Meaning from context Word parts Multiple meaning words

2nd Grade *continued*

Area	#	Common Core State Standard	Speech & Language Skills
L	5	Demonstrate understanding of word relationships and nuances in word meanings. a. Identify real-life connections between words and their use. b. Distinguish shades of meaning among closely related verbs and closely related adjectives.	Compare/contrast Verbs Adjectives
L	6	Use words and phrases acquired through conversations, reading and being read to, and responding to texts, including using adjectives and adverbs to describe.	Vocabulary Describe Adjectives Adverbs
OA	A1	Use addition and subtraction within 100 to solve one- and two-step word problems involving situations of adding to, taking from, putting together, taking apart, and comparing, with unknowns in all positions.	Concepts Compare/contrast Sequence
NBT	A4	Compare two three-digit numbers based on meanings of the hundreds, tens, and ones digits, using >, =, and < symbols to record the results of comparisons.	Compare/contrast
NBT	B5	Fluently add and subtract within 100 using strategies based on place value, properties of operations, and/or the relationship between addition and subtraction.	Compare/contrast
NBT	B7	Add and subtract within 1000, using concrete models or drawings and strategies based on place value, properties of operations, and/or the relationship between addition and subtraction; relate the strategy to a written method. Understand that in adding or subtracting three-digit numbers, one adds or subtracts hundreds and hundreds, tens and tens, ones and ones; and sometimes it is necessary to compose or decompose tens or hundreds.	Compare/contrast
NBT	B9	Explain why addition and subtraction strategies work, using place value and the properties of operations.	Infer/draw conclusions

2nd Grade *continued*

Area	#	Common Core State Standard	Speech & Language Skills
MD	A2	Measure the length of an object twice, using length units of different lengths for the two measurements; describe how the two measurements relate to the size of the unit chosen.	Describe
MD	D 10	Draw a picture graph and a bar graph (with single-unit scale) to represent a data set with up to four categories. Solve simple put-together, take-apart, and compare problems using information presented in a bar graph.	Compare/contrast Categorize
G	A3	Partition circles and rectangles into two, three, or four equal shares, describe the shares using the words halves, thirds, half of, a third of, etc., and describe the whole as two halves, three thirds, four fourths. Recognize that equal shares of identical wholes need not have the same shape.	Concepts Describe

3RD GRADE

Area	#	Common Core State Standard	Speech & Language Skills
RL RI	1	Ask and answer questions to demonstrate understanding of a text, referring explicitly to the text as the basis for the answers.	Ask questions Answer questions
RL	2	Recount stories, including fables, folktales, and myths from diverse cultures; determine the central message, lesson, or moral and explain how it is conveyed through key details in the text.	Retell Main idea Supporting details
RL	3	Describe characters in a story and explain how their actions contribute to the sequence of events.	Describe Cause/effect Sequence
RL	4	Determine the meaning of words and phrases as they are used in a text, distinguishing literal from nonliteral language.	Meaning from context Nonliteral language
RL	5	Refer to parts of stories, dramas, and poems when writing or speaking about a text, using terms such as chapter, scene, and stanza; describe how each successive part builds on earlier sections.	Describe Sequence
RL	6	Distinguish their own point of view from that of the narrator or those of the characters.	Compare/contrast Taking perspective of others
RL	7	Explain how specific aspects of a text's illustrations contribute to what is conveyed by the words in a story.	Compare/contrast
RI	2	Determine the main idea of a text; recount the key details and explain how they support the main idea.	Main idea Supporting details
RI	3	Describe the relationship between a series of historical events, scientific ideas or concepts, or steps in technical procedures in a text, using language that pertains to time, sequence, and cause/effect.	Concepts Sequence Cause/effect

3rd Grade *continued*

Area	#	Common Core State Standard	Speech & Language Skills
RI	4	Determine the meaning of general academic and domain-specific words and phrases in a text relevant to a *grade 3 topic or subject area.*	Meaning from context
RI	6	Distinguish their own point of view from that of the author of a text.	Taking perspective of others Compare/contrast
RI	9	Compare and contrast the most important points and key details presented in two texts on the same topic.	Compare/contrast Important versus unimportant details
W	1	Write opinion pieces on topics or texts, supporting a point of view with reasons. a. Introduce the topic or text they are writing about, state an opinion, and create an organizational structure that lists reasons. b. Provide reasons that support the opinion. c. Use linking words and phrases to connect opinion and reasons. d. Provide a concluding statement or section.	Main idea Fact/opinion Supporting details Sequence Conjunctions
W	2	Write informative/explanatory texts to examine a topic and convey ideas and information clearly. a. Introduce a topic and group related information together; include illustrations when useful to aiding comprehension. b. Develop the topic with facts, definitions, and details. c. Use linking words and phrases to connect ideas within categories of information. d. Provide a concluding statement or section.	Main idea Supporting details Categorize Sequence Conjunctions

3rd Grade *continued*

Area	#	Common Core State Standard	Speech & Language Skills
W	3	Write narratives to develop real or imagined experiences or events using effective technique, descriptive details, and clear event sequences. a. Establish a situation and introduce a narrator and/or characters; organize an event sequence that unfolds naturally. b. Use dialogue and descriptions of actions, thoughts, and feelings to develop experiences and events or show the response of characters to situations. c. Use temporal words and phrases to signal event order.	Concepts Describe Sequence Main idea Supporting details
W	5	With guidance and support from peers and adults, develop and strengthen writing as needed by planning, revising, and editing.	Syntax/morphology
W	6	With guidance and support from adults, use technology to produce and publish writing (using keyboarding skills) as well as to interact and collaborate with others.	Pragmatics
W	8	Recall information from experiences or gather information from print and digital sources; take brief notes on sources and sort evidence into provided categories.	Sort Categorize Retell
SL	1	Engage effectively in a range of collaborative discussions (one-to-one, in groups, and teacher-led) with diverse partners on *grade 3 topics and texts*, building on others' ideas and expressing their own clearly. a. Come to discussions prepared, having read or studied required material; explicitly draw on that preparation and other information known about the topic to explore ideas under discussion. b. Follow agreed-upon rules for discussions. c. Ask questions to check understanding of information presented, stay on topic, and link their comments to the remarks of others. d. Explain their own ideas and understanding in light of the discussion.	Pragmatics Ask questions

3rd Grade *continued*

Area	#	Common Core State Standard	Speech & Language Skills
SL	2	Determine the main ideas and supporting details of a text read aloud or information presented in diverse media and formats, including visually, quantitatively, and orally.	Main idea Supporting details
SL	3	Ask and answer questions about information from a speaker, offering appropriate elaboration and detail.	Ask questions Answer questions
SL	4	Report on a topic or text, tell a story, or recount an experience with appropriate facts and relevant, descriptive details, speaking clearly at an understandable pace.	Retell Main idea Supporting details Articulation/phonological processes
SL	6	Speak in complete sentences when appropriate to task and situation in order to provide requested detail or clarification.	Sentence construction Answer questions
L	1	Demonstrate command of the conventions of standard English grammar and usage when writing or speaking. a. Explain the function of nouns, pronouns, verbs, adjectives, and adverbs in general and their functions in particular sentences. b. Form and use regular and irregular plural nouns. c. Use abstract nouns. d. Form and use regular and irregular verbs. e. Form and use the simple verb tenses. f. Ensure subject-verb and pronoun-antecedent agreement. g. Form and use comparative and superlative adjectives and adverbs, and choose between them depending on what is to be modified. h. Use coordinating and subordinating conjunctions. i. Produce simple, compound, and complex sentences.	Nouns Pronouns Verbs Adjectives Adverbs Plurals Past tense Present tense Future tense Comparatives/Superlatives Conjunctions Sentence construction

3rd Grade *continued*

Area	#	Common Core State Standard	Speech & Language Skills
L	3	Use knowledge of language and its conventions when writing, speaking, reading, or listening.	Syntax/ morphology
L	4	Determine or clarify the meaning of unknown and multiple-meaning word and phrases based on *grade 3 reading and content*, choosing flexibly from a range of strategies. a. Use sentence-level context as a clue to the meaning of a word or phrase. b. Determine the meaning of the new word formed when a known affix is added to a word. c. Use a known root word as a clue to the meaning of an unknown word with the same root. d. Use glossaries or beginning dictionaries, both print and digital, determine or clarify the precise meaning of key words and phrases.	Meaning from context Word parts Multiple meaning words
L	5	Demonstrate understanding of word relationships and nuances in word meanings. a. Distinguish the literal and nonliteral meanings of words and phrases in context. b. Identify real-life connections between words and their use. c. Distinguish shades of meaning among related words that describe states of mind or degrees of certainty.	Describe Compare/contrast Meaning from context Nonliteral language
L	6	Acquire and use accurately grade-appropriate conversational, general academic, and domain-specific words and phrases, including those that signal spatial and temporal relationships.	Vocabulary Concepts
OA	C7	Fluently multiply and divide within 100, using strategies such as the relationship between multiplication and division or properties of operations. By the end of grade 3, know from memory all products of two one-digit numbers.	Compare/contrast

3rd Grade *continued*

Area	#	Common Core State Standard	Speech & Language Skills
OA	D8	Solve two-step word problems using the four operations. Represent these problems using equations with a letter standing for the unknown quantity. Assess the reasonableness of answers using mental computation and estimation strategies including rounding.	Sequence
NBT	A2	Fluently add and subtract within 1000 using strategies and algorithms based on place value, properties of operations, and/or the relationship between addition and subtraction.	Compare/contrast
NF	A3	Explain equivalence of fractions in special cases, and compare fractions by reasoning about their size. a. Understand two fractions as equivalent (equal) if they are the same size, or the same point on a number line. b. Recognize and generate simple equivalent fractions, e.g., $1/2 = 2/4$, $4/6 = 2/3$. Explain why the fractions are equivalent, e.g., by using a visual fraction model. d. Compare two fractions with the same numerator or the same denominator by reasoning about their size. Recognize that comparisons are valid only when the two fractions refer to the same whole. Record the results of comparisons with the symbols >, =, or <, and justify the conclusions.	Answer questions Compare/contrast
MD	B3	Draw a scaled picture graph and a scaled bar graph to represent a data set with several categories. Solve one- and two-step "how many more" and "how many less" problems using information presented in scaled bar graphs.	Concepts Categorize Sequence
G	A1	Understand that shapes in different categories may share attributes, and that the shared attributes can define a larger category. Recognize rhombuses, rectangles, and squares as examples of quadrilaterals, and draw examples of quadrilaterals that do not belong to any of these subcategories.	Categorize

		4TH GRADE	

Area	#	Common Core State Standard	Speech & Language Skills
RL	2	Determine a theme of a story, drama, or poem from details in the text; summarize the text.	Main idea Supporting details Summarize
RL	3	Describe in depth a character, setting, or event in a story or drama, drawing on specific details in the text.	Describe Narrative elements Supporting details
RL	4	Determine the meaning of words and phrases as they are used in a text, including those that allude to significant characters found in mythology.	Meaning from context
RL	5	Explain major differences between poems, drama, and prose, and refer to the structural elements of poems and drama when writing or speaking about a text.	Compare/contrast
RL	6	Compare and contrast the point of view from which different stories are narrated, including the difference between first- and third-person narrations.	Compare/contrast Taking perspective of others
RL	7	Make connections between the text of a story or drama and a visual or oral presentation of the text, identifying where each version reflects specific descriptions and directions in the text.	Compare/contrast Describe
RL	9	Compare and contrast the treatment of similar themes and topics and patterns of events in stories, myths, and traditional literature from different cultures.	Compare/contrast
RI	2	Determine the main idea of a text and explain how it is supported by key details; summarize the text.	Main idea Supporting details Summarize
RI	3	Explain events, procedures, ideas, or concepts in a historical, scientific, or technical text, including what happened and why, based on specific information in the text.	Describe Main idea Supporting details

4th Grade *continued*

Area	#	Common Core State Standard	Speech & Language Skills
RI	4	Determine the meaning of general academic and domain-specific words or phrases in a text relevant to a *grade 4 topic or subject area.*	Meaning from context
RI	5	Describe the overall structure of events, ideas, concepts, or information in a text or part of a text.	Describe
RI	6	Compare and contrast a firsthand and secondhand account of the same event or topic; describe the difference in focus and the information provided.	Compare/contrast
RI	7	Interpret information presented visually, orally, or quantitatively and explain how the information contributes to an understanding of the text in which it appears.	Cause/effect
RI	8	Explain how an author uses reasons and evidence to support particular points in a text.	Describe Supporting details
RI	9	Integrate information from two texts on the same topic in order to write or speak about the subject knowledgeably.	Compare/contrast
W	1	Write opinion pieces on topics or texts, supporting a point of view with reasons and information. a. Introduce a topic or text clearly, state an opinion, and create an organizational structure in which related ideas are grouped to support the writer's purpose. b. Provide reasons that are supported by facts and details. c. Link opinion and reasons using words and phrases. d. Provide a concluding statement or section related to the opinion presented.	Sequence Main idea Supporting details Fact/opinion

4th Grade *continued*

Area	#	Common Core State Standard	Speech & Language Skills
W	2	Write informative/explanatory texts to examine a topic and convey ideas and information clearly. a. Introduce a topic clearly and group related information in paragraphs and sections; include formatting, illustrations, and multimedia when useful to aiding comprehension. b. Develop the topic with facts, definitions, concrete details, quotations, or other information and examples related to the topic. c. Link ideas within categories of information using words and phrases. d. Use precise language and domain-specific vocabulary to inform about or explain the topic. e. Provide a concluding statement or section related to the information or explanation presented.	Categorize Sequence Main idea Supporting details Conjunctions
W	3	Write narratives to develop real or imagined experiences or events using effective technique, descriptive details, and clear event sequences. a. Orient the reader by establishing a situation and introducing a narrator and/or characters; organize an event sequence that unfolds naturally. b. Use dialogue and description to develop experiences and events or show the responses of characters to situations. c. Use a variety of transitional words and phrases to manage the sequence of events. d. Use concrete words and phrases and sensory details to convey experiences and events precisely. e. Provide a conclusion that follows from the narrated experiences or events.	Sequence Describe Retell Supporting details
W	5	With guidance and support from peers and adults, develop and strengthen writing as needed by planning, revising, and editing.	Syntax/morphology

4th Grade *continued*

Area	#	Common Core State Standard	Speech & Language Skills
W	6	With some guidance and support from adults, use technology, including the Internet, to produce and publish writing as well as to interact and collaborate with others; demonstrate sufficient command of keyboarding skills to type a minimum of one page in a single sitting.	Pragmatics
W	8	Recall relevant information from experiences or gather relevant information from print and digital sources; take notes and categorize information, and provide a list of sources.	Categorize Retell Important versus unimportant details
W	9	Draw evidence from literary or informational texts to support analysis, reflection, and research.	Supporting details
SL	1	Engage effectively in a range of collaborative discussions (one-on-one, in groups, and teacher-led) with diverse partners on *grade 4 topics and texts*, building on others' ideas and expressing their own clearly. a. Come to discussions prepared, having read or studied required material; explicitly draw on that preparation and other information known about the topic to explore ideas under discussion. b. Follow agreed-upon rules for discussions and carry out assigned roles. c. Pose and respond to specific questions to clarify or follow up on information, and make comments that contribute to the discussion and link to the remarks of others. d. Review key ideas expressed and explain their own ideas and understanding in light of the discussion.	Ask questions Answer questions Main idea Pragmatics
SL	2	Paraphrase portions of a text read aloud or information presented in diverse media and formats, including visually, quantitatively, and orally.	Summarize
SL	3	Identify the reasons and evidence a speaker provides to support particular points.	Supporting details

4th Grade *continued*

Area	#	Common Core State Standard	Speech & Language Skills
SL	4	Report on a topic or text, tell a story, or recount an experience in an organized manner, using appropriate facts and relevant, descriptive details to support main ideas or themes; speak clearly at an understandable pace.	Retell Main idea Supporting details Articulation/ phonological processes
L	1	Demonstrate command of the conventions of standard English grammar and usage when writing or speaking. a. Use relative pronouns (who, whose, whom, which, that) and relative adverbs (where, when, why). b. Form and use the progressive verb tenses. c. Use modal auxiliaries to convey various conditions. d. Order adjectives within sentences according to conventional patterns. e. Form and use prepositional phrases. f. Produce complete sentences, recognizing and correcting inappropriate fragments and run-ons.	Pronouns Present progressive Adjectives Sentence construction Prepositional phrases
L	3	Use knowledge of language and its conventions when writing, speaking, reading, or listening. a. Choose words and phrases to convey ideas precisely. c. Differentiate between contexts that call for formal English and situations where informal discourse is appropriate.	Syntax/ morphology

4th Grade *continued*

Area	#	Common Core State Standard	Speech & Language Skills
L	4	Determine or clarify the meaning of unknown and multiple-meaning words and phrases based on *grade 4 reading and content*, choosing flexibly from a range of strategies. a. Use content as a clue to the meaning of a word or phrase. b. Use common, grade-appropriate Greek and Latin affixes and roots as clues to the meaning of a word. c. Consult reference materials, both print and digital, to find the pronunciation and determine or clarify the precise meaning of key words and phrases.	Meaning from context Word parts Multiple meaning words
L	5	Demonstrate understanding of figurative language, word relationships, and nuances in word meanings. a. Explain the meaning of simple similes and metaphors in context. b. Recognize and explain the meaning of common idioms, adages, and proverbs. c. Demonstrate understanding of words by relating them to their opposites (antonyms) and to words with similar but not identical meanings (synonyms).	Meaning from context Figurative language Compare/contrast Antonyms Synonyms
L	6	Acquire and use accurately grade-appropriate general academic and domain-specific words and phrases, including those that signal precise actions, emotions, or states of being and that are basic to a particular topic.	Vocabulary Verbs Adjectives Adverbs
OA	A1	Interpret a multiplication equation as a comparison. Represent verbal statements of multiplicative comparisons as multiplication equations.	Compare/contrast

4th Grade *continued*

Area	#	Common Core State Standard	Speech & Language Skills
OA	A3	Solve multistep word problems posed with whole numbers and having whole-number answers using the four operations, including problems in which remainders must be interpreted. Represent these problems using equations with a letter standing for the unknown quantity. Assess the reasonableness of answers using mental computation and estimation strategies including rounding.	Sequence
OA	C5	Generate a number or shape pattern that follows a given rule. Identify apparent features of the pattern that were not explicit in the rule itself.	Sequence
NBT	A2	Read and write multidigit whole numbers using base-ten numerals, number names, and expanded form. Compare two multidigit numbers based on meanings of the digits in each place, using >, =, and < symbols to record the results of comparisons.	Compare/contrast
NBT	B6	Find whole-number quotients and remainders with up to four-digit dividends and one-digit divisors, using strategies based on place value, the properties of operations, and/or the relationship between multiplication and division. Illustrate and explain the calculation by using equations, rectangular arrays, and/or area models.	Compare/contrast
NF	A1	Explain why a fraction a/b is equivalent to a fraction $(n \times a)/(n \times b)$ by using visual fraction models, with attention to how the number and size of the parts differ even though the two fractions themselves are the same size. Use this principle to recognize and generate equivalent fractions.	Compare/contrast Infer/draw conclusions

4th Grade *continued*

Area	#	Common Core State Standard	Speech & Language Skills
NF	A2	Compare two fractions with different numerators and different denominators, for example, by creating common denominators or numerators, or by comparing to a benchmark fraction such as 1/2. Recognize that comparisons are valid only when the two fractions refer to the same whole. Record the results of comparisons with symbols >, =, or <, and justify the conclusions, e.g., by using a visual fraction model.	Compare/contrast Infer/draw conclusions
NF	B3	Understand a fraction a/b with $a > 1$ as a sum of fractions $1/b$. c. Add and subtract mixed numbers with like denominators, for example, by replacing each mixed number with an equivalent fraction, and/or by using properties of operations and the relationship between addition and subtraction.	Compare/contrast
NF	C7	Compare two decimals to hundredths by reasoning about their size. Recognize that comparisons are valid only when the two decimals refer to the same whole. Record the results of comparisons with the symbols >, =, or <, and justify the conclusions, for example, by using a visual model.	Compare/contrast Infer/draw conclusions
G	A2	Classify two-dimensional figures based on the presence or absence of parallel or perpendicular lines, or the presence or absence of angles of a specified size. Recognize right triangles as a category, and identify right triangles.	Categorize

5TH GRADE

Area	#	Common Core State Standard	Speech & Language Skills
RL RI	1	Quote accurately from a text when explaining what the text says explicitly and when drawing inferences from the text.	Describe Supporting details Infer/draw conclusions
RL	2	Determine a theme of a story, drama, or poem from details in the text, including how characters in a story or drama respond to challenges or how the speaker in a poem reflects upon a topic; summarize the text.	Main idea Supporting details Summarize
RL	3	Compare and contrast two or more characters, settings, or events in a story or drama, drawing on specific details in the text.	Compare/contrast Narrative elements
RL	4	Determine the meaning of words and phrases as they are used in a text, including figurative language such as metaphors and similes.	Meaning from context Figurative language
RL	5	Explain how a series of chapters, scenes, or stanzas fits together to provide the overall structure of a particular story, drama, or poem.	Describe
RL	6	Describe how a narrator's or speaker's point of view influences how events are described.	Describe Cause/effect Taking perspective of others
RL	9	Compare and contrast stories in the same genre on their approaches to similar themes and topics.	Compare/contrast
RI	2	Determine two or more main ideas of a text and explain how they are supported by key details; summarize the text.	Main idea Supporting details Summarize
RI	3	Explain the relationships or interactions between two or more individuals, events, ideas, or concepts in a historical, scientific, or technical text based on specific information in the text.	Compare/contrast

5th Grade *continued*

Area	#	Common Core State Standard	Speech & Language Skills
RI	4	Determine the meaning of general academic and domain-specific words and phrases in a text relevant to a *grade 5 topic or subject area*.	Meaning from context
RI	5	Compare and contrast the overall structure of events ideas, concepts, or information in two or more texts.	Compare/contrast
RI	6	Analyze multiple accounts of the same event or topic, noting important similarities and differences in the point of view they represent.	Compare/contrast Taking perspective of others
RI	7	Draw on information from multiple print or digital sources, demonstrating the ability to locate an answer to a question quickly or to solve a problem efficiently.	Answer questions Infer/draw conclusions
RI	8	Explain how an author uses reasons and evidence to support particular points in a text, identifying which reasons and evidence support which point(s).	Describe Supporting details
RI	9	Integrate information from several texts on the same topic in order to write or speak about the subject knowledgeably.	Compare/contrast
W	1	Write opinion pieces on topics or texts, supporting a point of view with reasons and information. a. Introduce a topic or text clearly, state an opinion, and create an organizational structure in which ideas are logically grouped to support the writer's purpose. b. Provide logically ordered reasons that are supported by facts and details. c. Link opinion and reasons using words, phrases, and clauses. d. Provide a concluding statement or section related to the opinion presented.	Categorize Sequence Main idea Supporting details Fact/opinion

5th Grade *continued*

Area	#	Common Core State Standard	Speech & Language Skills
W	2	Write informative/explanatory texts to examine a topic and convey ideas and information clearly. a. Introduce a topic clearly, provide a general observation and focus, and group related information logically; include formatting, illustrations, and multimedia when useful to aiding comprehension. b. Develop the topic with facts, definitions, concrete details, quotations, or other information and examples related to the topic. c. Link ideas within and across categories of information using words, phrases, and clauses. d. Use precise language and domain-specific vocabulary to inform about or explain the topic. e. Provide a concluding statement or section related to the information or explanation presented.	Describe Categorize Sequence Main idea Supporting details
W	3	Write narratives to develop real or imagined experiences or events using effective technique, descriptive details, and clear event sequences. a. Orient the reader by establishing a situation and introducing a narrator and/or characters; organize an event sequence that unfolds naturally. b. Use narrative techniques, such as dialogue, description, and pacing, to develop experiences and events or show the responses of characters to situations. c. Use a variety of transitional words, phrases, and clauses to manage the sequence of events. d. Use concrete words and phrases and sensory details to convey experiences and events precisely. e. Provide a conclusion that follows from the narrated experiences or events.	Describe Sequence Main idea Supporting details
W	5	With guidance and support from peers and adults, develop and strengthen writing as needed by planning, revising, editing, rewriting, or trying a new approach.	Syntax/ morphology

5th Grade *continued*

Area	#	Common Core State Standard	Speech & Language Skills
W	6	With some guidance and support from adults, use technology, including the Internet, to produce and publish writing as well as to interact and collaborate with others; demonstrate sufficient command of keyboarding skills to type a minimum of two pages in a single sitting.	Pragmatics
W	8	Recall relevant information from experiences or gather relevant information from print and digital sources; summarize or paraphrase information in notes and finished work, and provide a list of sources.	Important versus unimportant details Summarize
W	9	Draw evidence from literary or informational texts to support analysis, reflection, and research.	Supporting details
SL	1	Engage effectively in a range of collaborative discussions (one-to-one, in groups, and teacher-led) with diverse partners on *grade 5 topics and texts*, building on others' ideas and expressing their own clearly. a. Come to discussions prepared, having read or studied required material; explicitly draw on that preparation and other information known about the topic to explore ideas under discussion. b. Follow agreed-upon rules for discussions and carry out assigned roles. c. Pose and respond to specific questions by making comments that contribute to the discussion and elaborate on the remarks of others. d. Review the key ideas expressed and draw conclusions in light of information and knowledge gained from the discussions.	Ask questions Answer questions Main idea Infer/draw conclusions Pragmatics
SL	2	Summarize a written text read aloud or information presented in diverse media and formats, including visually, quantitatively, and orally.	Summarize
SL	3	Summarize the points a speaker makes and explain how each claim is supported by reasons and evidence.	Summarize Supporting details

5th Grade *continued*

Area	#	Common Core State Standard	Speech & Language Skills
SL	4	Report on a topic or text or present an opinion, sequencing ideas logically and using appropriate facts and relevant, descriptive details to support main ideas or themes; speak clearly at an understandable pace.	Sequence Main idea Supporting details Fact/opinion Articulation/ phonological processes
L	1	Demonstrate command of the conventions of standard English grammar and usage when writing or speaking. a. Explain the function of conjunctions, prepositions, and interjections in general and their function in particular sentences. b. Form and use the perfect verb tenses. c. Use verb tense to convey various times, sequences, states, and conditions. d. Recognize and correct inappropriate shifts in verb tense.	Conjunctions Concepts Past tense Present tense Future tense
L	3	Use knowledge of language and its conventions when writing, speaking, reading, or listening. b. Compare and contrast the varieties of English used in stories, dramas, or poems.	Compare/contrast Syntax/ morphology
L	4	Determine or clarify the meaning of unknown and multiple-meaning words and phrases based on *grade 5 reading and content*, choosing flexibly from a range of strategies. a. Use context as a clue to the meaning of a word or phrase. b. Use common grade-appropriate Greek and Latin affixes and roots as clues to the meaning of a word. c. Consult reference materials, both print and digital, to find the pronunciation and determine or clarify the precise meaning of key words and phrases.	Meaning from context Word parts Multiple meaning words

5th Grade *continued*

Area	#	Common Core State Standard	Speech & Language Skills
L	5	Demonstrate understanding of figurative language, word relationships, and nuances in word meanings. a. Interpret figurative language, including similes and metaphors, in context. b. Recognize and explain the meaning of common idioms, adages, and proverbs. c. Use the relationship between particular words to better understand each of the words.	Describe Compare/contrast Figurative language
L	6	Acquire and use accurately grade-appropriate general academic and domain-specific words and phrases, including those that signal contrast, addition, and other logical relationships.	Vocabulary
OA	B3	Generate two numerical patterns using two given rules. Identify apparent relationships between corresponding terms. Form ordered pairs consisting of corresponding terms from the two patterns, and graph the ordered pairs on a coordinate plane.	Compare/contrast
NBT	A2	Explain patterns in the number of zeros of the product when multiplying a number by powers of 10, and explain patterns in the placement of the decimal point when a decimal is multiplied or divided by a power of 10. Use whole-number exponents to denote powers of 10.	Compare/contrast
NBT	A3	Read, write, and compare decimals to thousandths. c. Compare two decimals to thousandths based on meanings of the digits in each place, using >, =, and < symbols to record the results of comparisons.	Compare/contrast
NBT	B6	Find whole-number quotients of whole numbers with up to four-digit dividends and two-digit divisors, using strategies based on place value, the properties of operations, and/or the relationship between multiplication and division. Illustrate and explain the calculation by using equations, rectangular arrays, and/or area models.	Compare/contrast

5th Grade *continued*

Area	#	Common Core State Standard	Speech & Language Skills
NBT	B7	Add, subtract, multiply, and divide decimals to hundredths, using concrete models or drawings and strategies based on place value, properties of operations, and/or the relationship between addition and subtraction; relate the strategy to a written method and explain the reasoning used.	Compare/contrast Infer/draw conclusions
NF	B4	Apply and extend previous understandings of multiplication to multiply a fraction or whole number by a fraction. a. Interpret the product (a/b) × q as a parts of a partition of q into b equal parts; equivalently, as the result of a sequence of operations a × q ÷ b.	Sequence
NF	B5	Interpret multiplication as scaling (resizing), by: a. Comparing the size of a product to the size of one factor on the basis of the size of the other factor, without performing the indicated multiplication. b. Explaining why multiplying a given number by a fraction greater than 1 results in a product greater than the given number (recognizing multiplication by whole numbers greater than 1 as a familiar case); explaining why multiplying a given number by a fraction less than 1 results in a product smaller than the given number; and relating the principle of fraction equivalence $a/b = (n \times a)/(n \times b)$ to the effect of multiplying a/b by 1.	Concepts Compare/contrast Infer/draw conclusions
G	B3	Understand that attributes belonging to a category of two-dimensional figures also belong to all subcategories of that category. For example, all rectangles have four right angles and squares are rectangles, so all squares have four right angles.	Categorize
G	B4	Classify two-dimensional figures in a hierarchy based on properties.	Categorize

6TH GRADE

Area	#	Common Core State Standard	Speech & Language Skills
RL RI	1	Cite textual evidence to support analysis of what the text says explicitly as well as inferences drawn from the text.	Supporting details Infer/draw conclusions
RL	2	Determine a theme or central idea of a text and how it is conveyed through particular details; provide a summary of the text distinct from personal opinions or judgments.	Main idea Supporting details Summarize Fact/opinion
RL	3	Describe how a particular story's or drama's plot unfolds in a series of episodes as well as how the characters respond or change as the plot moves toward a resolution.	Describe Cause/effect
RL	4	Determine the meaning of words and phrases as they are used in a text, including figurative and connotative meanings; analyze the impact of a specific word choice on meaning and tone.	Meaning from context Compare/contrast Figurative language
RL	5	Analyze how a particular sentence, chapter, scene, or stanza fits into the overall structure of a text and contributes to the development of the theme, setting, or plot.	Cause/effect Main idea
RL	6	Explain how an author develops the point of view of the narrator or speaker in a text.	Describe Taking perspective of others
RL	7	Compare and contrast the experience of reading a story, drama, or poem to listening to or viewing an audio, video, or live version of the text, including contrasting what they "see" and "hear" when reading the text to what they perceive when they listen or watch.	Compare/contrast

6th Grade *continued*

Area	#	Common Core State Standard	Speech & Language Skills
RL	9	Compare and contrast texts in different forms or genres in terms of their approaches to similar themes and topics.	Compare/contrast
RI	2	Determine a central idea of a text and how it is conveyed through particular details; provide a summary of the text distinct from personal opinions or judgments.	Main idea Supporting details Summarize Fact/opinion
RI	4	Determine the meaning of words and phrases as they are used in a text, including figurative, connotative, and technical meanings.	Meaning from context Figurative language
RI	5	Analyze how a particular sentence, paragraph, chapter, or section fits into the overall structure of a text and contributes to the development of the ideas.	Cause/effect
RI	6	Determine an author's point of view or purpose in a text and explain how it is conveyed in the text.	Describe Main idea Supporting details
RI	7	Integrate information presented in different media or formats as well as in words to develop a coherent understanding of a topic or issue.	Main idea Supporting details
RI	8	Trace and evaluate the argument and specific claims in a text, distinguishing claims that are supported by reasons and evidence from claims that are not.	Compare/contrast Supporting details
RI	9	Compare and contrast one author's presentation of events with that of another.	Compare/contrast

6th Grade *continued*

Area	#	Common Core State Standard	Speech & Language Skills
W	1	Write arguments to support claims with clear reasons and relevant evidence. a. Introduce claim(s) and organize the reasons and evidence clearly. b. Support claim(s) with clear reasons and relevant evidence, using credible sources and demonstrating an understanding of the topic or text. c. Use words, phrases, and clauses to clarify the relationships among claim(s) and reasons. e. Provide a concluding statement or section that follows from the argument presented.	Categorize Sequence Main idea Supporting details
W	2	Write informative/explanatory texts to examine a topic and convey ideas, concepts, and information through the selection, organization, and analysis of relevant content. a. Introduce a topic; organize ideas, concepts, and information, using strategies such as definition, classification, comparison/contrast, and cause/effect; include formatting, graphics, and multimedia when useful to aiding comprehension. b. Develop the topic with relevant facts, definitions, concrete details, quotations, or other information and examples. d. Use precise language and domain-specific vocabulary to inform about or explain the topic. f. Provide a concluding statement or section that follows from the information or explanation presented.	Describe Categorize Compare/contrast Sequence Main idea Supporting details Cause/effect

6th Grade *continued*

Area	#	Common Core State Standard	Speech & Language Skills
W	3	Write narratives to develop real or imagined experiences or events using effective technique, relevant descriptive details, and well-structured event sequences. 　a. Engage and orient the reader by establishing a context and introducing a narrator and/or characters; organize an event sequence that unfolds naturally and logically. 　b. Use narrative techniques, such as dialogue, pacing, and description, to develop experiences, events, and/or characters. 　c. Use a variety of transition words, phrases, and clauses to convey sequence and signal shifts from one time frame or setting to another. 　d. Use precise words and phrases, relevant descriptive details, and sensory language to convey experiences and events. 　e. Provide a conclusion that follows from the narrated experiences or events.	Describe Sequence Main idea Supporting details
W	5	With some guidance and support from peers and adults, develop and strengthen writing as needed by planning, revising, editing, rewriting, or trying a new approach.	Syntax/morphology Pragmatics
W	6	Use technology, including the Internet, to produce and publish writing as well as to interact and collaborate with others; demonstrate sufficient command of keyboarding skills to type a minimum of three pages in a single sitting.	Pragmatics
W	7	Conduct short research projects to answer a question, drawing on several sources and refocusing the inquiry when appropriate.	Answer questions
W	8	Gather relevant information from multiple print and digital sources; assess the credibility of each source; and quote or paraphrase the data and conclusions of others while avoiding plagiarism and providing basic bibliographic information for sources.	Important versus unimportant details Summarize

6th Grade *continued*

Area	#	Common Core State Standard	Speech & Language Skills
W	9	Draw evidence from literary or informational texts to support analysis, reflection, and research.	Supporting details
SL	1	Engage effectively in a range of collaborative discussions (one-on-one, in groups, and teacher-led) with diverse partners *on grade 6 topics, texts, and issues,* building on others' ideas and expressing their own clearly. a. Come to discussions prepared, having read or studied required material; explicitly draw on that preparation by referring to evidence on the topic, text, or issue to probe and reflect on ideas under discussion. b. Follow rules for collegial discussions, set specific goals and deadlines, and define individual roles as needed. c. Pose and respond to specific questions with elaboration and detail by making comments that contribute to the topic, text, or issue under discussion. d. Review the key ideas expressed and demonstrate understanding of multiple perspectives through reflection and paraphrasing.	Ask questions Answer questions Summarize Main idea Supporting details Pragmatics
SL	2	Interpret information presented in diverse media and formats and explain how it contributes to a topic, text, or issue under study.	Describe
SL	3	Delineate a speaker's argument and specific claims, distinguishing claims that are supported by reasons and evidence from claims that are not.	Compare/contrast Supporting details

6th Grade *continued*

Area	#	Common Core State Standard	Speech & Language Skills
SL	4	Present claims and findings, sequencing ideas logically and using pertinent descriptions, facts, and details to accentuate main ideas or themes; use appropriate eye contact, adequate volume, and clear pronunciation.	Describe Sequence Main idea Supporting details Fact/opinion Nonverbal cues Articulation/ phonological processes
SL	6	Adapt speech to a variety of contexts and tasks, demonstrating command of formal English when indicated or appropriate.	Syntax/ morphology

L	1	Demonstrate command of the conventions of standard English grammar and usage when writing or speaking.
		
		   a. Ensure that pronouns are in the proper case (subjective, objective, possessive).
		   b. Use intensive pronouns.
		   c. Recognize and correct inappropriate shifts in pronoun number and person.
		   d. Recognize and correct vague pronouns (i.e., ones with unclear or ambiguous antecedents).
			Pronouns

L	3	Use knowledge of language and its conventions when writing, speaking, reading, or listening.	Syntax/ morphology

6th Grade *continued*

Area	#	Common Core State Standard	Speech & Language Skills
L	4	Determine or clarify the meaning of unknown and multiple-meaning words and phrases based on *grade 6 reading and content*, choosing flexibly from a range of strategies. a. Use context as a clue to the meaning of a word or phrase. b. Use common, grade-appropriate Greek or Latin affixes and roots as clues to the meaning of a word. c. Consult reference materials, both print and digital, to find the pronunciation of a word or determine or clarify its precise meaning or its part of speech. d. Verify the preliminary determination of the meaning of a word or phrase.	Meaning from context Word parts Multiple meaning words
L	5	Demonstrate understanding of figurative language, word relationships, and nuances in word meanings. a. Interpret figures of speech in context. b. Use the relationship between particular words to better understand each of the words. c. Distinguish among the connotations (associations) of words with similar denotations (definitions).	Compare/contrast Figurative language
L	6	Acquire and use accurately grade-appropriate general academic and domain-specific words and phrases; gather vocabulary knowledge when considering a word or phrase important to comprehension and expression.	Vocabulary
RP	A1	Understand the concept of a ratio and use ratio language to describe a ratio relationship between two quantities.	Describe Compare/contrast

6th Grade *continued*

Area	#	Common Core State Standard	Speech & Language Skills
RP	A3	Use ratio and rate reasoning to solve real-world and mathematical problems, for example, by reasoning about tables of equivalent ratios, tape diagrams, double number line diagrams, or equations. a. Make tables of equivalent ratios relating quantities with whole-number measurements, find missing values in the tables, and plot the pairs of values on the coordinate plane. Use tables to compare ratios.	Compare/contrast
NS	C7	Understand ordering and absolute value of rational numbers. d. Distinguish comparisons of absolute value from statements about order.	Compare/contrast
EE	B5	Understand solving an equation or inequality as a process of answering a question: which values from a specified set, if any, make the equation or inequality true? Use substitution to determine whether a given number in a specified set makes an equation or inequality true.	Answer questions
EE	C9	Use variables to represent two quantities in a real-world problem that change in relationship to one another; write an equation to express one quantity, thought of as the dependent variable, in terms of the other quantity, thought of as the independent variable. Analyze the relationship between the dependent and independent variables using graphs and tables, and relate these to the equation.	Compare/contrast

6th Grade *continued*

Area	#	Common Core State Standard	Speech & Language Skills
SP	B5	Summarize numerical data sets in relation to their context, such as by: b. Describing the nature of the attribute under investigation, including how it was measured and its units of measurement. c. Giving quantitative measures of center (median and/or mean) and variability (interquartile range and/or mean absolute deviation), as well as describing any overall pattern and any striking deviations from the overall pattern with reference to the context in which the data were gathered.	Describe Sequence
RH	2	Determine the central ideas or information of a primary or secondary source; provide an accurate summary of the source distinct from prior knowledge of opinions.	Main idea Summarize Fact/opinion
RH	3	Identify key steps in a text's description of a process related to history/social studies.	Sequence Important versus unimportant details
RH	4	Determine the meaning of words and phrases as they are used in a text, including vocabulary specific to domains related to history/social studies.	Meaning from context
RH	5	Describe how a text presents information.	Describe
RH	8	Distinguish among fact, opinion, and reasoned judgment in a text.	Fact/opinion
RH	9	Analyze the relationship between a primary and secondary source on the same topic.	Compare/contrast
RST	2	Determine the central ideas or conclusions of a text; provide an accurate summary of the text distinct from prior knowledge or opinions.	Summarize Main idea Infer/draw conclusions Fact/opinion

6th Grade *continued*

Area	#	Common Core State Standard	Speech & Language Skills
RST	3	Follow precisely a multistep procedure when carrying out experiments, taking measurements, or performing technical tasks.	Sequence
RST	4	Determine the meaning of symbols, key terms, and other domain-specific words and phrases as they are used in a specific scientific or technical context relevant to *grades 6 to 8 texts and topics*.	Meaning from context
RST	8	Distinguish among facts, reasoned judgment based on research findings, and speculation in a text.	Fact/opinion
RST	9	Compare and contrast the information gained from experiments, simulations, video, or multimedia sources with that gained from reading a text on the same topic.	Compare/contrast

7TH GRADE

Area	#	Common Core State Standard	Speech & Language Skills
RL RI	1	Cite several pieces of textual evidence to support analysis of what the text says explicitly as well as inferences drawn from the text.	Supporting details Infer/draw conclusions
RL	2	Determine a theme or central idea of a text and analyze its development over the course of the text; provide an objective summary of the text.	Main idea Sequence Summarize
RL	3	Analyze how particular elements of a story or drama interact.	Compare/contrast
RL	4	Determine the meaning of words and phrases as they are used in a text, including figurative and connotative meanings; analyze the impact of rhymes and other repetitions of sounds on a specific verse or stanza of a poem or section of a story or drama.	Meaning from context Figurative language
RL	5	Analyze how a drama's or poem's form or structure contributes to its meaning.	Cause/effect
RL	6	Analyze how an author develops and contrasts the points of view of different characters or narrators in a text.	Compare/contrast Taking perspective of others
RL	7	Compare and contrast a written story, drama, or poem to its audio, filmed, staged, or multimedia version, analyzing the effects or techniques unique to each medium.	Compare/contrast
RL	9	Compare and contrast a fictional portrayal of a time, place, or character and a historical account of the same period as a means of understanding how authors of fiction use or alter history.	Compare/contrast Narrative elements
RI	2	Determine two or more central ideas in a text and analyze their development over the course of the text; provide an objective summary of the text.	Main idea Sequence Summarize

7th Grade *continued*

Area	#	Common Core State Standard	Speech & Language Skills
RI	3	Analyze the interactions between individuals, events, and ideas in a text.	Compare/contrast
RI	4	Determine the meaning of words and phrases as they are used in a text, including figurative, connotative, and technical meanings; analyze the impact of a specific word choice on meaning and tone.	Meaning from context Figurative language
RI	5	Analyze the structure an author uses to organize a text, including how the major sections contribute to the whole and to the development of the ideas.	Sequence
RI	6	Determine an author's point of view or purpose in a text and analyze how the author distinguishes his or her position from that of others.	Main idea Compare/contrast
RI	7	Compare and contrast a text to an audio, video, or multimedia version of the text, analyzing each medium's portrayal of the subject.	Compare/contrast
RI	8	Trace and evaluate the argument and specific claims in a text, assessing whether the reasoning is sound and the evidence is relevant and sufficient to support the claims.	Supporting details
RI	9	Analyze how two or more author's writing about the same topic shape their presentations of key information by emphasizing different evidence or advancing different interpretations of facts.	Compare/contrast
W	1	Write arguments to support claims with clear reasons and relevant evidence. a. Introduce claim(s), acknowledge alternate or opposing claims, and organize the reasons and evidence logically. b. Support claim(s) with logical reasoning and relevant evidence, using accurate, credible sources and demonstrating an understanding of the topic or text. e. Provide a concluding statement or section that follows from and supports the argument presented.	Categorize Sequence Main idea Supporting details Taking perspective of others

7th Grade *continued*

Area	#	Common Core State Standard	Speech & Language Skills
W	2	Write informative/explanatory texts to examine a topic and convey ideas, concepts, and information through the selection, organization, and analysis of relevant content. a. Introduce a topic clearly, previewing what is to follow; organize ideas, concepts, and information, using strategies such as definition, classification, comparison/contrast, and cause/effect; include formatting, graphics, and multimedia when useful to aiding comprehension. b. Develop the topic with relevant facts, definitions, concrete details, quotations, or other information and examples. d. Use precise language and domain-specific vocabulary to inform about or explain the topic. f. Provide a concluding statement or section that follows from and supports the information or explanation presented.	Describe Categorize Sequence Compare/contrast Cause/effect Main idea Supporting details
W	3	Write narratives to develop real or imagined experiences or events using effective technique, relevant descriptive details, and well-structured event sequences. a. Engage and orient the reader by establishing a context and point of view and introducing a narrator and/or characters; organize an event sequence that unfolds naturally and logically. b. Use narrative techniques, such as dialogue, pacing, and description, to develop experiences, events, and/or characters. c. Use a variety of transition words, phrases, and clauses to convey sequence and signal shifts from one time frame or setting to another. d. Use precise words and phrases, relevant descriptive details, and sensory language to capture the action and convey experiences and events. e. Provide a conclusion that follows from and reflects on the narrated experiences or events.	Describe Sequence Main idea

7th Grade *continued*

Area	#	Common Core State Standard	Speech & Language Skills
W	4	Produce clear and coherent writing in which the development, organization, and style are appropriate to task, purpose, and audience.	Categorize Sequence
W	5	With some guidance and support from peers and adults, develop and strengthen writing as needed by planning, revising, editing, rewriting, or trying a new approach, focusing on how well purpose and audience have been addressed.	Syntax/ morphology Pragmatics
W	6	Use technology, including the Internet, to produce and publish writing and link to and cite sources as well as to interact and collaborate with others, including linking to and citing sources.	Pragmatics
W	7	Conduct short research projects to answer a question, drawing on several sources and generating additional related, focused questions for further research and investigation.	Ask questions Answer questions
W	8	Gather relevant information from multiple print and digital sources, using search terms effectively; assess the credibility and accuracy of each source; and quote or paraphrase the data and conclusions of others while avoiding plagiarism and following a standard format for citation.	Sequence Important versus unimportant details Summarize
W	9	Draw evidence from literary or informational texts to support analysis, reflection, and research.	Supporting details

7th Grade *continued*

Area	#	Common Core State Standard	Speech & Language Skills
SL	1	Engage effectively in a range of collaborative discussions (one-to-one, in groups, and teacher-led) with diverse partners *on grade 7 topics, texts, and issues*, building on others' ideas and expressing their own clearly. a. Come to discussions prepared, having read or researched material under study; explicitly draw on that preparation by referring to evidence on the topic, text, or issue to probe and reflect on ideas under discussion. b. Follow rules for collegial discussions, track progress toward specific goals and deadlines, and define individual roles as needed. c. Pose questions that elicit elaboration and respond to others' questions and comments with relevant observations and ideas that bring the discussion back on topic as needed. d. Acknowledge new information expressed by others and, when warranted, modify their own views.	Ask questions Answer questions Main idea Supporting details Pragmatics
SL	2	Analyze the main ideas and supporting details presented in diverse media and formats and explain how the ideas clarify a topic, text, or issue under study.	Main idea Supporting details
SL	3	Delineate a speaker's argument and specific claims, evaluating the soundness of the reasoning and the relevance and sufficiency of the evidence.	Supporting details
SL	4	Present claims and findings, emphasizing salient points in a focused, coherent manner with pertinent descriptions, facts, details, and examples; use appropriate eye contact, adequate volume, and clear pronunciation.	Describe Important versus unimportant details Nonverbal cues Articulation/ phonological processes

7th Grade *continued*

Area	#	Common Core State Standard	Speech & Language Skills
L	1	Demonstrate command of the conventions of standard English grammar and usage when writing or speaking. a. Explain the function of phrases and clauses in general and their function in specific sentences. b. Choose among simple, compound, complex, and compound-complex sentences to signal differing relationships among ideas. c. Place phrases and clauses within a sentence, recognizing and correcting misplaced and dangling modifiers.	Sentence construction
L	3	Use knowledge of language and its conventions when writing, speaking, reading, or listening.	Syntax/ morphology
L	4	Determine or clarify the meaning of unknown and multiple-meaning words and phrases based on *grade 7 reading and content*, choosing flexibly from a range of strategies. a. Use context as a clue to the meaning of a word or phrase. b. Use common, grade-appropriate Greek or Latin affixes and roots as clues to the meaning of a word. c. Consult general and specialized reference materials, both print and digital, to find the pronunciation of a word or determine or clarify its precise meaning or its part of speech. d. Verify the preliminary determination of the meaning of a word or phrase.	Meaning from context Word parts Multiple meaning words
L	5	Demonstrate understanding of figurative language, word relationships, and nuances in word meanings. a. Interpret figures of speech in context. b. Use the relationship between particular words to better understand each of the words. c. Distinguish among the connotations (associations) of words with similar denotations (definitions).	Compare/contrast Figurative language

7th Grade *continued*

Area	#	Common Core State Standard	Speech & Language Skills
L	6	Acquire and use accurately grade-appropriate general academic and domain-specific words and phrases; gather vocabulary knowledge when considering a word or phrase important to comprehension and expression.	Vocabulary
RP	A2	Recognize and represent proportional relationships between quantities. b. Identify the constant of proportionality (unit rate) in tables, graphs, equations, diagrams, and verbal descriptions of proportional relationships. d. Explain what a point (x, y) on the graph of a proportional relationship means in terms of the situation, with special attention to the points $(0, 0)$ and $(1, r)$ where r is the unit rate.	Describe Compare/contrast
NS	A1	Apply and extend previous understandings of addition and subtraction to add and subtract rational numbers; represent addition and subtraction on a horizontal or vertical number line diagram. a. Describe situations in which opposite quantities combine to make 0.	Describe
EE	B3	Solve multistep real-life and mathematical problems posed with positive and negative rational numbers in any form (whole numbers, fractions, and decimals), using tools strategically. Apply properties of operations to calculate with numbers in any form; convert between forms as appropriate; and assess the reasonableness of answers using mental computation and estimation strategies.	Sequence

7th Grade *continued*

Area	#	Common Core State Standard	Speech & Language Skills
EE	B4	Use variables to represent quantities in a real-world or mathematical problem, and construct simple equations and inequalities to solve problems by reasoning about the quantities. a. Solve word problems leading to equations of the form $px + q = r$ and $p(x + q) = r$, where p, q, and r are specific rational numbers. Solve equations of these forms fluently. Compare an algebraic solution to an arithmetic solution, identifying the sequence of the operations used in each approach.	Sequence Compare/contrast
G	A3	Describe the two-dimensional figures that result from slicing three-dimensional figures, as in plane sections of right rectangular prisms and right rectangular pyramids.	Describe
SP	A2	Use data from a random sample to draw inferences about a population with an unknown characteristic of interest. Generate multiple samples (or simulated samples) of the same size to gauge the variation in estimates or predictions.	Infer/draw conclusions
SP	B4	Use measures of center and measures of variability for numerical data from random samples to draw informal comparative inferences about two populations.	Compare/contrast Infer/draw conclusions
SP	C6	Approximate the probability of a chance event by collecting data on the chance process that produces it and observing its long-run relative frequency, and predict the approximate relative frequency given the probability.	Predict
SP	C7	Develop a probability model and use it to find probabilities of events. Compare probabilities from a model to observed frequencies; if the agreement is not good, explain possible sources of the discrepancy.	Describe Compare/contrast
RH	2	Determine the central ideas or information of a primary or secondary source; provide an accurate summary of the source distinct from prior knowledge or opinions.	Main idea Supporting details Fact/opinion

7th Grade *continued*

Area	#	Common Core State Standard	Speech & Language Skills
RH	3	Identify key steps in a text's description of a process related to history/social studies.	Sequence Important versus unimportant details
RH	4	Determine the meaning of words and phrases as they are used in a text, including vocabulary specific to domains related to history/social studies.	Meaning from context
RH	5	Describe how a text presents information.	Describe
RH	8	Distinguish among fact, opinion, and reasoned judgment in a text.	Fact/opinion
RH	9	Analyze the relationship between a primary and secondary source on the same topic.	Compare/contrast
RST	2	Determine the central ideas or conclusions of a text; provide an accurate summary of the text distinct from prior knowledge or opinions.	Summarize Main idea Infer/draw conclusions Fact/opinion
RST	3	Follow precisely a multistep procedure when carrying out experiments, taking measurements, or performing technical tasks.	Sequence
RST	4	Determine the meaning of symbols, key terms, and other domain-specific words and phrases as they are used in a specific scientific or technical context relevant to *grades 6 to 8 texts and topics*.	Meaning from context
RST	8	Distinguish among facts, reasoned judgment based on research findings, and speculation in a text.	Fact/opinion
RST	9	Compare and contrast the information gained from experiments, simulations, video, or multimedia sources with that gained from reading a text on the same topic.	Compare/contrast

8TH GRADE

Area	#	Common Core State Standard	Speech & Language Skills
RL RI	1	Cite the textual evidence that most strongly supports an analysis of what the text says explicitly as well as inferences drawn from the text.	Supporting details Infer/draw conclusions
RL	2	Determine a theme or central idea of a text and analyze its development over the course of the text, including its relationship to the characters, setting, and plot; provide an objective summary of the text.	Main idea Supporting details Summarize Narrative elements
RL	3	Analyze how particular lines of dialogue or incidents in a story or drama propel the action, reveal aspects of a character, or provoke a decision.	Cause/effect
RL	4	Determine the meaning of words and phrases as they are used in a text, including figurative and connotative meanings; analyze the impact of specific word choices on meaning and tone, including analogies or allusions to other texts.	Meaning from context Figurative language
RL	5	Compare and contrast the structure of two or more texts and analyze how the differing structure of each text contributes to its meaning and style.	Compare/contrast
RL	6	Analyze how differences in the points of view of the characters and the audience or reader create such effects as suspense or humor.	Compare/contrast Taking perspective of others
RL	7	Analyze the extent to which a filmed or live production of a story or drama stays faithful to or departs from the text or script, evaluating the choices made by the director or actors.	Compare/contrast
RL	9	Analyze how a modern work of fiction draws on themes, patterns of events, or character types from myths, traditional stories, or religious works such as the Bible, including describing how the material is rendered new.	Describe Compare/contrast Main idea

8th Grade *continued*

Area	#	Common Core State Standard	Speech & Language Skills
RI	2	Determine a central idea of a text and analyze its development over the course of the text, including its relationship to supporting ideas; provide an objective summary of the text.	Sequence Summarize Main idea Supporting details
RI	3	Analyze how a text makes connections among and distinctions between individuals, ideas, or events.	Compare/contrast
RI	4	Determine the meaning of words and phrases as they are used in a text, including figurative, connotative, and technical meanings; analyze the impact of a specific word choice on meaning and tone, including analogies or allusions to other texts.	Meaning from context Figurative language
RI	5	Analyze in detail the structure of a specific paragraph in a text, including the role of particular sentences in developing and refining a key concept.	Main idea Supporting details
RI	6	Determine an author's point of view or purpose in a text and analyze how the author acknowledges and responds to conflicting evidence or viewpoints.	Main idea Taking perspective of others
RI	7	Evaluate the advantages and disadvantages of using different mediums to present a particular topic or idea.	Compare/contrast
RI	8	Delineate and evaluate the argument and specific claims in a text, assessing whether the reasoning is sound and the evidence is relevant and sufficient; recognize when irrelevant evidence is introduced.	Supporting details
RI	9	Analyze a case in which two or more texts provide conflicting information on the same topic and identify where the texts disagree on matters of fact or interpretation.	Compare/contrast Fact/opinion

8th Grade *continued*

Area	#	Common Core State Standard	Speech & Language Skills
W	1	Write arguments to support claims with clear reasons and relevant evidence a. Introduce claim(s), acknowledge and distinguish the claim(s) from alternate or opposing claims, and organize the reasons and evidence logically. b. Support claim(s) with logical reasoning and relevant evidence, using accurate, credible sources and demonstrating an understanding of the topic or text. c. Use words, phrases, and clauses to create cohesion and clarify the relationships among claim(s), counterclaims, reasons, and evidence. e. Provide a concluding statement or section that follows from and supports the argument presented.	Categorize Sequence Main idea Supporting details Taking perspective of others
W	2	Write informative/explanatory texts to examine a topic and convey ideas, concepts, and information through the selection, organization, and analysis of relevant content. a. Introduce a topic clearly, previewing what is to follow; organize ideas, concepts, and information into broader categories; include formatting (e.g., headings), graphics (e.g., charts, tables), and multimedia when useful to aiding comprehension. b. Develop the topic with relevant, well-chosen facts, definitions, concrete details, quotations, or other information and examples. d. Use precise language and domain-specific vocabulary to inform about or explain the topic. f. Provide a concluding statement or section that follows from and supports the information or explanation presented.	Describe Categorize Sequence Main idea Supporting details

8th Grade *continued*

Area	#	Common Core State Standard	Speech & Language Skills
W	3	Write narratives to develop real or imagined experiences or events using effective technique, relevant descriptive details, and well-structured event sequences. a. Engage and orient the reader by establishing a context and point of view and introducing a narrator and/or characters; organize an event sequence that unfolds naturally and logically. b. Use narrative techniques, such as dialogue, pacing, description, and reflection, to develop experiences, events, and/or characters. c. Use a variety of transition words, phrases, and clauses to convey sequence, signal shifts from one time frame or setting to another, and show the relationships among experiences and events. d. Use precise words and phrases, relevant descriptive details, and sensory language to capture the action and convey experiences and events. e. Provide a conclusion that follows from and reflects on the narrated experiences or events.	Describe Sequence Main idea Supporting details
W	4	Produce clear and coherent writing in which the development, organization, and style are appropriate to task, purpose, and audience.	Categorize Sequence
W	5	With some guidance and support from peers and adults, develop and strengthen writing as needed by planning, revising, editing, rewriting, or trying a new approach, focusing on how well purpose and audience have been addressed.	Syntax/ morphology Pragmatics
W	6	Use technology, including the Internet, to produce and publish writing and present the relationships between information and ideas efficiently as well as to interact and collaborate with others.	Compare/contrast Supporting details Pragmatics

8th Grade *continued*

Area	#	Common Core State Standard	Speech & Language Skills
W	7	Conduct short research projects to answer a question (including a self-generated question), drawing on several sources and generating additional related, focused questions that allow for multiple avenues of exploration.	Ask questions Answer questions
W	8	Gather relevant information from multiple print and digital sources, using search terms effectively; assess the credibility and accuracy of each source; and quote or paraphrase the data and conclusions of others while avoiding plagiarism and following a standard format for citation.	Sequence Important versus unimportant details Summarize
W	9	Draw evidence from literary or informational texts to support analysis, reflection, and research.	Supporting details
SL	1	Engage effectively in a range of collaborative discussions (one-on-one, in groups, and teacher-led) with diverse partners on *grade 8 topics, texts, and issues,* building on others' ideas and expressing their own clearly. a. Come to discussions prepared, having read or researched material under study; explicitly draw on that preparation by referring to evidence on the topic, text, or issue to probe and reflect on ideas under discussion. b. Follow rules for collegial discussions and decision-making, track progress toward specific goals and deadlines, and define individual roles as needed. c. Pose questions that connect the ideas of several speakers and respond to others' questions and comments with relevant evidence, observations, and ideas. d. Acknowledge new information expressed by others and, when warranted, qualify or justify their own views in light of the evidence presented.	Ask questions Answer questions Main idea Supporting details Pragmatics

8th Grade *continued*

Area	#	Common Core State Standard	Speech & Language Skills
SL	2	Analyze the purpose of information presented in diverse media and formats and evaluate the motives behind its presentation.	Main idea Supporting details
SL	3	Delineate a speaker's argument and specific claims, evaluating the soundness of the reasoning and the relevance and sufficiency of the evidence and identifying when irrelevant evidence is introduced.	Supporting details
SL	4	Present claims and findings, emphasizing salient points in a focused, coherent manner with relevant evidence, sound valid reasoning, and well-chosen details; use appropriate eye contact, adequate volume, and clear pronunciation.	Important versus unimportant details Supporting details Nonverbal cues Articulation/ phonological processes
SL	6	Adapt speech to a variety of contexts and tasks, demonstrating command of formal English when indicated or appropriate.	Syntax/ morphology

L	1	Demonstrate command of the conventions of standard English grammar and usage when writing or speaking.
		  a. Explain the function of verbals (gerunds, participles, infinitives) in general and their function in particular sentences.
		  b. Form and use verbs in the active and passive voice.
		  c. Form and use verbs in the indicative, imperative, interrogative, conditional, and subjunctive mood.
		  d. Recognize and correct inappropriate shifts in verb voice and mood.
			Verbs

L	3	Use knowledge of language and its conventions when writing, speaking, reading, or listening. a. Use verbs in the active and passive voice and in the conditional and subjunctive mood to achieve particular effects.	Verbs

8th Grade *continued*

Area	#	Common Core State Standard	Speech & Language Skills
L	4	Determine or clarify the meaning of unknown and multiple-meaning words and phrases based on *grade 8 reading and content*, choosing flexibly from a range of strategies. a. Use context as a clue to the meaning of a word or phrase. b. Use common, grade-appropriate Greek or Latin affixes and roots as clues to the meaning of a word. c. Consult general and specialized reference materials, both print and digital, to find the pronunciation of a word or determine or clarify its precise meaning or its part of speech. d. Verify the preliminary determination of the meaning of a word or phrase.	Meaning from context Word parts Multiple meaning words Compare/contrast
L	5	Demonstrate understanding of figurative language, word relationships, and nuances in word meanings. a. Interpret figures of speech in context. b. Use the relationship between particular words to better understand each of the words. c. Distinguish among the connotations (associations) of words with similar denotations (definitions).	Compare/contrast Figurative language
L	6	Acquire and use accurately grade-appropriate general academic and domain-specific words and phrases; gather vocabulary knowledge when considering a word or phrase important to comprehension and expression.	Vocabulary
NS	A2	Use rational approximations of irrational numbers to compare the size of irrational numbers, locate them approximately on a number line diagram, and estimate the value of expressions.	Compare/contrast
EE	B5	Graph proportional relationships, interpreting the unit rate as the slope of the graph. Compare two different proportional relationships represented in different ways.	Compare/contrast

8th Grade *continued*

Area	#	Common Core State Standard	Speech & Language Skills
F	A2	Compare properties of two functions each represented in a different way (algebraically, graphically, numerically in tables, or by verbal descriptions).	Compare/contrast
F	B4	Construct a function to model a linear relationship between two quantities. Determine the rate of change and initial value of the function from a description of a relationship or from two (x, y) values, including reading these from a table or from a graph. Interpret the rate of change and initial value of a linear function in terms of the situation it models, and in terms of its graph or a table of values.	Compare/contrast
F	B5	Describe qualitatively the functional relationship between two quantities by analyzing a graph. Sketch a graph that exhibits the qualitative features of a function that has been described verbally.	Describe
G	A2	Understand that a two-dimensional figure is congruent to another if the second can be obtained from the first by a sequence of rotations, reflections, and translations; given two congruent figures, describe a sequence that exhibits the congruence between them.	Describe Sequence
G	A4	Understand that a two-dimensional figure is similar to another if the second can be obtained from the first by a sequence of rotations, reflections, translations, and dilations; given two similar two-dimensional figures, describe a sequence that exhibits the similarity between them.	Describe Sequence Compare/contrast
G	B6	Explain a proof of the Pythagorean Theorem and its converse.	Describe

8th Grade *continued*

Area	#	Common Core State Standard	Speech & Language Skills
SP	A4	Understand that patterns of association can also be seen in bivariate categorical data by displaying frequencies and relative frequencies in a two-way table. Construct and interpret a two-way table summarizing data on two categorical variables collected from the same subjects. Use relative frequencies calculated for rows or columns to describe possible association between the two variables.	Describe Summarize
RH	2	Determine the central ideas or information of a primary or secondary source; provide an accurate summary of the source distinct from prior knowledge or opinions.	Main idea Supporting details Fact/opinion
RH	3	Identify key steps in a text's description of a process related to history/social studies.	Sequence
RH	4	Determine the meaning of words and phrases as they are used in a text, including vocabulary specific to domains related to history/social studies.	Meaning from context
RH	5	Describe how a text presents information.	Describe
RH	8	Distinguish among fact, opinion, and reasoned judgment in a text.	Fact/opinion
RH	9	Analyze the relationship between a primary and secondary source on the same topic.	Compare/contrast
RST	2	Determine the central ideas or conclusions of a text; provide an accurate summary of the text distinct from prior knowledge or opinions.	Summarize Main idea Infer/draw conclusions Fact/opinion
RST	3	Follow precisely a multistep procedure when carrying out experiments, taking measurements, or performing technical tasks.	Sequence

8th Grade *continued*

Area	#	Common Core State Standard	Speech & Language Skills
RST	4	Determine the meaning of symbols, key terms, and other domain-specific words and phrases as they are used in a specific scientific or technical context relevant to *grades 6 to 8 texts and topics.*	Meaning from context
RST	8	Distinguish among facts, reasoned judgment based on research findings, and speculation in a text.	Fact/opinion
RST	9	Compare and contrast the information gained from experiments, simulations, video, or multimedia sources with that gained from reading a text on the same topic.	Compare/contrast

9TH–10TH GRADE

Area	#	Common Core State Standard	Speech & Language Skills
RL RI	1	Cite strong and thorough textual evidence to support analysis of what the text says explicitly as well as inferences drawn from the text.	Supporting details Infer/draw conclusions
RL	2	Determine a theme or central idea of a text and analyze in detail its development over the course of the text, including how it emerges and is shaped and refined by specific details; provide an objective summary of the text.	Sequence Summarize Main idea Supporting details
RL	3	Analyze how complex characters develop over the course of a text, interact with other characters, and advance the plot or develop the theme.	Sequence Main idea
RL	4	Determine the meaning of words and phrases as they are used in the text, including figurative and connotative meanings; analyze the cumulative impact of specific word choices on meaning and tone.	Meaning from context Figurative language
RL	5	Analyze how an author's choices concerning how to structure a text, order events within it, and manipulate time create such effects as mystery, tension, or surprise.	Sequence Cause/effect
RL	6	Analyze a particular point of view or cultural experience reflected in a work of literature from outside the United States, drawing on a wide reading of world literature.	Taking perspective of others
RL	7	Analyze the representation of a subject or a key scene in two different artistic mediums, including what is emphasized or absent in each treatment.	Compare/contrast
RI	2	Determine a central idea of a text and analyze in detail its development over the course of the text, including how it emerges and is shaped and refined by specific details; provide an objective summary of the text.	Sequence Summarize Main idea Supporting details

9th–10th Grade *continued*

Area	#	Common Core State Standard	Speech & Language Skills
RI	3	Analyze how the author unfolds an analysis or series of ideas or events, including the order in which the points are made, how they are introduced and developed, and the connections that are drawn between them.	Sequence Supporting details Compare/contrast
RI	4	Determine the meaning of words and phrases as they are used in a text, including figurative, connotative, and technical meanings; analyze the cumulative impact of specific word choices on meaning and tone.	Meaning from context Figurative language
RI	6	Determine an author's point of view or purpose in a text and analyze how an author uses rhetoric to advance that point of view or purpose.	Main idea Supporting details Taking perspective of others
RI	7	Analyze various accounts of a subject told in different mediums, determining which details are emphasized in each account.	Compare/contrast Supporting details
RI	8	Delineate and evaluate the argument and specific claims in a text, assessing whether the reasoning is valid and the evidence is relevant and sufficient; identify false statements and fallacious reasoning.	Supporting details

9th–10th Grade *continued*

Area	#	Common Core State Standard	Speech & Language Skills
W	1	Write arguments to support claims in an analysis of substantive topics or texts, using valid reasoning and relevant and sufficient evidence. a. Introduce precise claim(s), distinguish the claim(s) from alternate or opposing claims, and create an organization that establishes clear relationships among claim(s), counterclaims, reasons, and evidence. b. Develop claim(s) and counterclaims fairly, supplying evidence for each while pointing out the strengths and limitations of both in a manner that anticipates the audience's knowledge level and concerns. c. Use words, phrases, and clauses to link the major sections of the text, create cohesion, and clarify the relationships between claim(s) and reasons, between reasons and evidence, and between claim(s) and counterclaims. e. Provide a concluding statement or section that follows from and supports the argument presented.	Categorize Sequence Main idea Supporting details Compare/contrast Taking perspective of others
W	2	Write informative/explanatory texts to examine and convey complex ideas, concepts, and information clearly and accurately through the effective selection, organization, and analysis of content. a. Introduce a topic; organize complex ideas, concepts, and information to make important connections and distinctions; include formatting, graphics, and multimedia when useful to aiding comprehension. b. Develop the topic with well-chosen, relevant, and sufficient facts, extended definitions, concrete details, quotations, or other information and examples appropriate to the audience's knowledge of the topic. f. Provide a concluding statement or section that follows from and supports the information or explanation presented.	Categorize Sequence Main idea Supporting details

9th–10th Grade *continued*

Area	#	Common Core State Standard	Speech & Language Skills
W	3	Write narratives to develop real or imagined experiences or events using effective technique, well-chosen details, and well-structured event sequences. a. Engage and orient the reader by setting out a problem, situation, or observation, establishing one or multiple point(s) of view, and introducing a narrator and/or characters; create a smooth progression of experiences or events. b. Use narrative techniques, such as dialogue, pacing, description, reflection, and multiple plot lines, to develop experiences, events, and/or characters. c. Use a variety of techniques to sequence events so that they build on one another to create a coherent whole. d. Use precise words and phrases, telling details, and sensory language to convey a vivid picture of the experiences, events, setting, and/or characters. e. Provide a conclusion that follows from and reflects on what is experienced, observed, or resolved over the course of the narrative.	Describe Sequence Main idea Supporting details Taking perspective of others
W	4	Produce clear and coherent writing in which the development, organization, and style are appropriate to task, purpose, and audience.	Categorize Sequence
W	5	Develop and strengthen writing as needed by planning, revising, editing, rewriting, or trying a new approach, focusing on addressing what is most significant for a specific purpose and audience.	Syntax/morphology
W	7	Conduct short, as well as more sustained research projects, to answer a question (including a self-generated question) or solve a problem; narrow or broaden the inquiry when appropriate; synthesize multiple sources on the subject, demonstrating understanding of the subject under investigation.	Ask questions Answer questions Problem solve

9th–10th Grade *continued*

Area	#	Common Core State Standard	Speech & Language Skills
W	8	Gather relevant information from multiple authoritative print and digital sources, using advanced searches effectively; assess the usefulness of each source in answering the research question; integrate information into the text selectively to maintain the flow of ideas, avoiding plagiarism and following a standard format for citation.	Sequence Important versus unimportant details Summarize Supporting details
W	9	Draw evidence from literary or informational texts to support analysis, reflection, and research.	Supporting details
SL	1	Initiate and participate effectively in a range of collaborative discussions (one-on-one, in groups, and teacher-led) with diverse partners on *grades 9 to 10 topics, texts, and issues*, building on others' ideas and expressing their own clearly and persuasively. a. Come to discussions prepared, having read and researched material under study; explicitly draw on that preparation by referring to evidence from texts and other research on the topic or issue to stimulate a thoughtful, well-reasoned exchange of ideas. b. Work with peers to set rules for collegial discussions and decision-making, clear goals and deadlines, and individual roles as needed. c. Propel conversations by posing and responding to questions that relate the current discussion to broader themes or larger ideas; actively incorporate others into the discussion; and clarify, verify, or challenge ideas and conclusions. d. Respond thoughtfully to diverse perspectives, summarize points of agreement and disagreement, and, when warranted, qualify or justify their own views and understanding and make new connections in light of the evidence and reasoning presented.	Ask questions Answer questions Summarize Main idea Supporting details Pragmatics

9th–10th Grade *continued*

Area	#	Common Core State Standard	Speech & Language Skills
SL	2	Integrate multiple sources of information presented in diverse media or formats evaluating the credibility and accuracy of each source.	Compare/contrast
SL	3	Evaluate a speaker's point of view, reasoning, and use of evidence and rhetoric, identifying any fallacious reasoning or exaggerated or distorted evidence.	Supporting details Taking perspective of others
SL	4	Present information, findings, and supporting evidence clearly, concisely, and logically such that listeners can follow the line of reasoning and the organization, development, substance, and style are appropriate to purpose, audience, and task.	Sequence Supporting details
SL	6	Adapt speech to a variety of contexts and tasks, demonstrating command of formal English when indicated or appropriate.	Syntax/morphology
L	1	Demonstrate command of the conventions of standard English grammar and usage when writing or speaking. b. Use various types of phrases (noun, verb, adjectival, adverbial, participial, prepositional, absolute) and clauses (independent, dependent; noun, relative, adverbial) to convey specific meanings and add variety and interest to writing or presentations.	Nouns Verbs Adjectives Adverbs Prepositional phrases

9th–10th Grade *continued*

Area	#	Common Core State Standard	Speech & Language Skills
L	4	Determine or clarify the meaning of unknown and multiple-meaning words and phrases based on *grades 9 to 10 reading and content*, choosing flexibly from a range of strategies. a. Use context as a clue to the meaning of a word or phrase. b. Identify or correctly use patterns of word changes that indicate different meanings or parts of speech. c. Consult general and specialized reference materials, both print and digital, to find the pronunciation of a word or determine or clarify its precise meaning, its part of speech, or its etymology. d. Verify the preliminary determination of the meaning of a word or phrase.	Meaning from context Multiple meaning words Compare/contrast
L	5	Demonstrate understanding of figurative language, word relationships, and nuances in word meanings. a. Interpret figures of speech in context and analyze their role in the text. b. Analyze nuances in the meaning of words with similar denotations.	Compare/contrast Figurative language
L	6	Acquire and use accurately general academic and domain-specific words and phrases, sufficient for reading, writing, speaking, and listening at the college and career readiness level; demonstrate independence in gathering vocabulary knowledge when considering a word or phrase important to comprehension or expression.	Vocabulary
RH	2	Determine the central ideas or information of a primary or secondary source; provide an accurate summary of how key events of ideas develop over the course of the text.	Main idea Important versus unimportant details Summarize

9th–10th Grade *continued*

Area	#	Common Core State Standard	Speech & Language Skills
RH	3	Analyze in detail a series of events described in a text; determine whether earlier events caused later ones or simply preceded them.	Cause/effect Sequence
RH	4	Determine the meaning of words and phrases as they are used in a text, including vocabulary describing political, social, or economic aspects of history/social studies.	Meaning from context
RH	6	Compare the point of view of two or more authors for how they treat the same or similar topics, including which details they include and emphasize in their respective accounts.	Compare/contrast Taking perspective of others
RH	8	Assess the extent to which the reasoning and evidence in a text support the author's claims.	Supporting details
RH	9	Compare and contrast treatments of the same topic in several primary and secondary sources.	Compare/contrast
RST	2	Determine the central ideas or conclusions of a text; trace the text's explanation or depiction of a complex process, phenomenon, or concept; provide an accurate summary of the text.	Summarize Main idea Infer/draw conclusions
RST	3	Follow precisely a complex multistep procedure when carrying out experiments, taking measurements, or performing technical tasks, attending to special cases or exceptions defined in the text.	Sequence
RST	4	Determine the meaning of symbols, key terms, and other domain-specific words and phrases as they are used in a specific scientific or technical context relevant to *grades 9 to 10 texts and topics.*	Meaning from context
RST	5	Analyze the structure of the relationships among concepts in a text, including relationships among key terms.	Compare/contrast

9th–10th *continued*

Area	#	Common Core State Standard	Speech & Language Skills
RST	8	Assess the extent to which the reasoning and evidence in a text support the author's claim or a recommendation for solving a scientific or technical problem.	Infer/draw conclusions Problem solve
RST	9	Compare and contrast findings presented in a text to those from other sources (including their own experiments), noting when the findings support or contradict previous explanations or accounts.	Compare/contrast

11TH–12TH GRADE

Area	#	Common Core State Standard	Speech & Language Skills
RL RI	1	Cite strong and thorough textual evidence to support analysis of what the text says explicitly as well as inferences drawn from the text, including determining where the text leaves matters uncertain.	Supporting details Infer/draw conclusions
RL	2	Determine two or more themes or central ideas of a text and analyze their development over the course of the text, including how they interact and build on one another to produce a complex account; provide an objective summary of the text.	Sequence Summarize Main idea Supporting details
RL	3	Analyze the impact of the author's choices regarding how to develop and relate elements of a story or drama.	Supporting details
RL	4	Determine the meaning of words and phrases as they are used in a text, including figurative and connotative meanings; analyze the impact of specific word choices on meaning and tone, including words with multiple meanings or language that is particularly fresh, engaging, or beautiful. (Include Shakespeare as well as other authors.)	Meaning from context Multiple meaning words Figurative language
RL	5	Analyze how an author's choices concerning how specific parts of a text contribute to its overall structure and meaning as well as its aesthetic impact.	Meaning from context
RL	6	Analyze a case in which grasping a point of view requires distinguishing what is directly stated in a text from what is really meant.	Infer/draw conclusions Taking perspective of others
RL	7	Analyze multiple interpretations of a story, drama, or poem, evaluating how each version interprets the source text.	Compare/contrast

11th–12th Grade *continued*

Area	#	Common Core State Standard	Speech & Language Skills
RL	9	Demonstrate knowledge of eighteenth-, nineteenth-, and early-twentieth-century foundational works of American literature, including how two or more texts from the same period treat similar themes or topics.	Compare/contrast
RI	2	Determine two or more central ideas of a text and analyze their development over the course of the text, including how they interact and build on one another to provide a complex analysis; provide an objective summary of the text.	Sequence Summarize Main idea Supporting details
RI	3	Analyze a complex set of ideas or sequence of events and explain how specific individuals, ideas, or events interact and develop over the course of the text.	Sequence
RI	4	Determine the meaning of words and phrases as they are used in a text, including figurative, connotative, and technical meanings; analyze how an author uses and refines the meaning of a key term or terms over the course of a text.	Meaning from context Figurative language
RI	5	Analyze and evaluate the effectiveness of the structure an author uses in his or her exposition or argument, including whether the structure makes points clear, convincing, and engaging.	Supporting details
RI	6	Determine an author's point of view or purpose in a text in which the rhetoric is particularly effective, analyzing how style and content contribute to the power, persuasiveness, or beauty of the text.	Supporting details Taking perspective of others
RI	7	Integrate and evaluate multiple sources of information presented in different media or formats as well as in words in order to address a question or solve a problem.	Answer questions Compare/contrast Problem solve

11th–12th Grade *continued*

Area	#	Common Core State Standard	Speech & Language Skills
W	1	Write arguments to support claims in an analysis of substantive topics or texts, using valid reasoning and relevant and sufficient evidence. a. Introduce precise, knowledgeable claim(s), establish the significance of the claim(s), distinguish the claim(s) from alternate or opposing claims, and create an organization that logically sequences claim(s), counterclaims, reasons, and evidence. b. Develop claim(s) and counterclaims fairly and thoroughly, supplying the most relevant evidence for each while pointing out the strengths and limitations of both in a manner that anticipates the audience's knowledge level, concerns, values, and possible biases. c. Use words, phrases, and clauses as well as varied syntax to link the major sections of the text, create cohesion, and clarify the relationships between claim(s) and reasons, between reasons and evidence, and between claim(s) and counterclaims. e. Provide a concluding statement or section that follows from and supports the argument presented.	Describe Sequence Main idea Supporting details Compare/contrast Taking perspective of others Syntax/morphology

11th–12th Grade *continued*

Area	#	Common Core State Standard	Speech & Language Skills
W	2	Write informative/explanatory texts to examine and convey complex ideas, concepts, and information clearly and accurately through the effective selection, organization, and analysis of content. a. Introduce a topic; organize complex ideas, concepts, and information so that each new element builds on that which precedes it to create a unified whole; include formatting, graphics, and multimedia when useful to aiding comprehension. b. Develop the topic thoroughly by selecting the most significant and relevant facts, extended definitions, concrete details, quotations, or other information and examples appropriate to the audience's knowledge of the topic. c. Use appropriate and varied transitions and syntax to link the major sections of the text, create cohesion, and clarify the relationships among complex ideas and concepts. d. Use precise language, domain-specific vocabulary, and techniques such as metaphor, simile, and analogy to manage the complexity of the topic. f. Provide a concluding statement or section that follows from and supports the information or explanation presented.	Describe Categorize Sequence Main idea Supporting details Figurative language

11th–12th Grade *continued*

Area	#	Common Core State Standard	Speech & Language Skills
W	3	Write narratives to develop real or imagined experiences or events using effective technique, well-chosen details, and well-structured event sequences. a. Engage and orient the reader by setting out a problem, situation, or observation and its significance, establishing one or multiple point(s) of view, and introducing a narrator and/or characters; create a smooth progression of experiences or events. b. Use narrative techniques, such as dialogue, pacing, description, reflection, and multiple plot lines, to develop experiences, events, and/or characters. c. Use a variety of techniques to sequence events so that they build on one another to create a coherent whole and build toward a particular tone and outcome. d. Use precise words and phrases, telling details, and sensory language to convey a vivid picture of the experiences, events, setting, and/or characters. e. Provide a conclusion that follows from and reflects on what is experienced, observed, or resolved over the course of the narrative.	Describe Sequence Main idea Supporting details Taking perspective of others
W	4	Produce clear and coherent writing in which the development, organization, and style are appropriate to task, purpose, and audience.	Categorize Sequence
W	5	Develop and strengthen writing as needed by planning, revising, editing, rewriting, or trying a new approach, focusing on addressing what is most significant for a specific purpose and audience.	Syntax/morphology
W	7	Conduct short as well as more sustained research projects to answer a question (including a self-generated question) or solve a problem; narrow or broaden the inquiry when appropriate; synthesize multiple sources on the subject, demonstrating understanding of the subject under investigation.	Ask questions Answer questions Problem solve

11th–12th Grade *continued*

Area	#	Common Core State Standard	Speech & Language Skills
W	8	Gather relevant information from multiple authoritative print and digital sources, using advanced searches effectively; assess the strengths and limitations of each source in terms of the task, purpose, and audience; integrate information into the text selectively to maintain the flow of ideas, avoiding plagiarism and overreliance on any one source and following a standard format for citation.	Sequence Important versus unimportant details Summarize
W	9	Draw evidence from literary or informational texts to support analysis, reflection, and research.	Supporting details
SL	1	Initiate and participate effectively in a range of collaborative discussions (one-on-one, in groups, and teacher-led) with diverse partners on *grades 11 to 12 topics, texts, and issues*, building on others' ideas and expressing their own clearly and persuasively. a. Come to discussions prepared, having read and researched material under study; explicitly draw on that preparation by referring to evidence from texts and other research on the topic or issue to stimulate a thoughtful, well-reasoned exchange of ideas. b. Work with peers to promote civil, democratic discussions and decision-making, set clear goals and deadlines, and establish individual roles as needed. c. Propel conversations by posing and responding to questions that probe reasoning and evidence; ensure a hearing for a full range of positions on a topic or issue; clarify, verify, or challenge ideas and conclusions; and promote divergent and creative perspectives. d. Respond thoughtfully to diverse perspectives; synthesize comments, claims, and evidence made on all sides of an issue; resolve contradictions when possible; and determine what additional information or research is required to deepen the investigation or complete the task.	Ask questions Answer questions Main idea Supporting details Pragmatics

11th–12th Grade *continued*

Area	#	Common Core State Standard	Speech & Language Skills
SL	2	Integrate multiple sources of information presented in diverse formats and media in order to make informed decisions and solve problems, evaluating the credibility and accuracy of each source and noting any discrepancies among the data.	Compare/contrast Supporting details Problem solve
SL	3	Evaluate a speaker's point of view, reasoning, and use of evidence and rhetoric, assessing the stance, premises, links among ideas, word choice, points of emphasis, and tone used.	Taking perspective of others
SL	4	Present information, findings, and supporting evidence, conveying a clear and distinct perspective, such that listeners can follow the line of reasoning, alternative or opposing perspectives are addressed, and the organization, development, substance, and style are appropriate to purpose, audience, and a range of formal and informal tasks.	Sequence Supporting details Taking perspective of others
SL	6	Adapt speech to a variety of contexts and tasks, demonstrating command of formal English when indicated or appropriate.	Syntax/ morphology
L	1	Demonstrate command of the conventions of standard English grammar and usage when writing or speaking.	Syntax/ morphology
L	3	Apply knowledge of language to understand how language functions in different contexts, to make effective choices for meaning or style, and to comprehend more fully when reading or listening. a. Vary syntax for effect, consulting references for guidance as needed; apply an understanding of syntax to the study of complex texts when reading.	Syntax/ morphology

11th–12th Grade *continued*

Area	#	Common Core State Standard	Speech & Language Skills
L	4	Determine or clarify the meaning of unknown and multiple-meaning words and phrases based on *grades 11 to 12 reading and content*, choosing flexibly from a range of strategies. a. Use context as a clue to the meaning of a word or phrase. b. Identify or correctly use patterns of word changes that indicate different meanings or parts of speech. c. Consult general and specialized reference materials, both print and digital, to find the pronunciation of a word or determine or clarify its precise meaning, its part of speech, or its etymology, or its standard usage. d. Verify the preliminary determination of the meaning of a word or phrase.	Meaning from context Multiple meaning words
L	5	Demonstrate understanding of figurative language, word relationships, and nuances in word meanings. a. Interpret figures of speech in context and analyze their role in the text. b. Analyze nuances in the meaning of words with similar denotations.	Compare/contrast Figurative language
L	6	Acquire and use accurately general academic and domain-specific words and phrases, sufficient for reading, writing, speaking, and listening at the college and career readiness level; demonstrate independence in gathering vocabulary knowledge when considering a word or phrase important to comprehension or expression.	Vocabulary
RH	2	Determine the central ideas or information of a primary or secondary source; provide an accurate summary that makes clear the relationships among the key details and ideas.	Main idea Supporting details Summarize Compare/contrast

11th–12th Grade *continued*

Area	#	Common Core State Standard	Speech & Language Skills
RH	3	Evaluate various explanations for actions or events and determine which explanation best accords with textual evidence, acknowledging where the text leaves matters uncertain.	Compare/contrast
RH	4	Determine the meaning of words and phrases as they are used in a text, including analyzing how an author uses and refines the meaning of a key term over the course of a text.	Meaning from context
RH	7	Integrate and evaluate multiple sources of information presented in diverse formats and media in order to address a question or solve a problem.	Answer questions Problem solve
RST	2	Determine the central ideas or conclusions of a text; summarize complex concepts, processes, or information presented in a text by paraphrasing them in simpler but still accurate terms.	Summarize Main idea Infer/draw conclusions
RST	3	Follow precisely a complex multistep procedure when carrying out experiments, taking measurements, or performing technical tasks; analyze the specific results based on explanations in the text.	Sequence
RST	4	Determine the meaning of symbols, key terms, and other domain-specific words and phrases as they are used in a specific scientific or technical context relevant to *grades 11 to 12 texts and topics.*	Meaning from context
RST	5	Analyze how the text structures information or ideas into categories or hierarchies, demonstrating understanding of the information or ideas.	Categorize
RST	9	Synthesize information from a range of sources into a coherent understanding of a process, phenomenon, or concept, resolving conflicting information when possible.	Summarize

3

Prerequisite Skills and Steps to Mastery

The speech-language skills in this chapter are organized into the following areas:

- Vocabulary

- Questions

- Summarize

- Main Idea and Details

- Critical Thinking

- Pragmatics

- Syntax and Morphology

- Articulation and Phonological Processes

These areas were selected as they are major domains of language development and common areas requiring speech-language intervention. Each area includes a brief explanation followed by a listing of *Prerequisite Skills* and corresponding *Steps to Mastery*.

An index of prerequisite skills has been provided in Table 3–1 so the SLP can easily locate the skills identified in Chapters 1 and 2.

Table 3–1. Index of Prerequisite Skills

Prerequisite Skill	Speech-Language Area
Adjectives	Vocabulary
Adverbs	Vocabulary
Answer factual questions	Critical Thinking
Antonyms/synonyms	Vocabulary
Articles	Syntax and Morphology
Ask a question	Questions
Categorize	Vocabulary
Cause/effect	Questions Critical Thinking
Comparatives/superlatives	Vocabulary Syntax and Morphology
Compare/contrast	Vocabulary Critical Thinking

Answer questions:
  Yes/no
  What
  Where
  Who
  When
  Why
  How
	Questions
	Main Idea and Details
	Summarize

Concepts	Vocabulary
Conjunctions	Syntax and Morphology
Conversational repairs	Pragmatics
Describe	Vocabulary
Fact/opinion	Critical Thinking
Figurative language	Critical Thinking Pragmatics
Future tense	Syntax and Morphology

Table 3–1. *continued*

Prerequisite Skill	Speech-Language Area
Greetings/farewells	Pragmatics
Identify own emotions	Pragmatics
Identify what information is needed	Questions
Important versus unimportant details	Main Idea and Details Summarize Critical Thinking
Infer/draw conclusions	Questions Main Idea and Details Critical Thinking
Initiating conversation	Pragmatics
Main idea	Main Idea and Details
Match	Vocabulary
Meaning from context	Vocabulary
Multiple meaning words	Vocabulary
Narrative elements	Questions Summarize
Negation	Vocabulary
Nonliteral language	Critical Thinking Pragmatics
Nonverbal cues	Pragmatics
Nouns	Vocabulary
Past tense	Syntax and Morphology
Plurals	Syntax and Morphology
Possessives	Syntax and Morphology
Predict	Critical Thinking
Prepositional phrases	Syntax and Morphology
Present progressive	Syntax and Morphology
Present tense	Syntax and Morphology

continues

Table 3–1. *continued*

Prerequisite Skill	Speech-Language Area
Problem solve	Critical Thinking Pragmatics
Pronouns	Vocabulary Syntax and Morphology
Protesting	Pragmatics
Request for object or action	Pragmatics
Request help, information, clarification	Pragmatics
Responding	Pragmatics
Retell	Summarize
Sentence construction	Syntax and Morphology
Sequence	Main Idea and Details Summarize Critical Thinking
Sequence Concepts	Summarize
Sort	Vocabulary
Summarize	Summarize
Supporting details	Main Idea and Details
Taking perspective of others	Pragmatics
Telling versus asking	Questions
Topic maintenance, joining in, exiting, ending	Pragmatics
Verbs	Vocabulary

The *Prerequisite Skills* are not aligned with a specific age or grade level. Any student at any age, grade, or level of functioning could have or lack any of the prerequisite skills indicated. Students may also display splinter skills, meaning that there are gaps in the developmental sequence of learning a skill. If splinter skills exist, identify those that are lacking to fill in the gaps. While the *Prerequisite Skills* are generally listed in a hierarchy, some develop simultaneously with differing degrees of difficulty. For example, the skill of cause/effect is listed before infer/draw conclusions, but these skills, at the most basic level, develop simultaneously. Skills that have already been mastered at one grade will continue to develop as a student moves on to the upper grades. One example of this would be *Main Idea and Details*. In the lower grades, a student needs to identify a stated main idea. In the upper grades, a student needs to infer the main idea and provide supporting details.

The *Steps to Mastery* outline what is necessary for mastery of the corresponding *Prerequisite Skill*. Any of these steps can be developed into IEP goals. Each step can be an entry point or an ending point for a student. The entry point is the step where the student is currently functioning. This is where interventions should begin. The goal(s) placed in an IEP should be the ending point of what the student can reasonably attain in the timeframe of the IEP. In the *Steps to Mastery*, the steps often include object, picture, picture scene, sentence, paragraph, and then, story. This represents a hierarchy from easiest to most difficult. It does not represent the activities or strategies that could be used in therapy. Even if a state or school system has not adopted the Common Core State Standards, the *Steps to Mastery* will be very useful in focusing on the skills the SLPs commonly teach.

Once the SLP has identified which *Step to Mastery* is the student's ending point, an IEP goal needs to be written. Proceed to Chapter 4 for information on how to transform the *Steps to Mastery* into IEP goals.

VOCABULARY

Vocabulary forms the foundation for all language skills. A student's vocabulary will typically reflect their experience and background knowledge. Vocabulary terms are not learned by a certain age or grade; instead, the extent of the vocabulary depends on the experiences and exposures of the individual child (Beck, Kucan, & McKeown, 2013). Without a foundation of vocabulary terms (e.g., nouns, verbs, pronouns, adjectives, concepts), it will be very difficult for a student to reach any of the prerequisites for the other language skill areas covered in this book.

There are different opinions as to what the role of the speech-language pathologist (SLP) should be in regard to vocabulary instruction. Should the SLP teach grade-level/content vocabulary, which requires memorization of definitions? Should a goal be written for defining vocabulary words since this is often an issue for students with language impairments once they reach the upper elementary grades? Should the SLP focus on concepts?

Research supports the fact that vocabulary has a strong relationship with reading comprehension and general intelligence (Loraine, 2008). Vocabulary has been identified by the National Reading Panel as one of the five major elements for reading. Therefore, explicit vocabulary instruction is an important aspect of classroom instruction (National Reading Technical Assistance Center [NRTAC], 2010). The SLP can support this instruction in therapy by providing students the opportunity to experience vocabulary. It is important that this exposure is provided in context and is functional for individual students (Banotai, 2010).

In our professional opinion, the SLP's role in regard to vocabulary instruction and the writing of IEP goals should be based on skills, not memorization. There are students who need to be taught linguistic concepts and specific vocabulary. Once it has been established that a student has a core receptive and expressive vocabulary, including basic concepts, the SLP should ensure that the student has the strategies to learn the meanings of new or unknown words. If a student is having difficulty defining words used in his or her grade-level curriculum, it is essential to discover why. Is the student better able to identify the meaning when given choices? Does he or she have difficulty using context clues to help determine the meaning of words? If the student can identify the meaning of a word, can he or she explain it in their own words? Or, does the student have difficulties with the skill of describing?

SLPs should carefully choose vocabulary terms during intervention in order to teach word-learning strategies and language skills. Terms to consider should not include only curriculum vocabulary but also high-frequency word lists, Tier 2 vocabulary, and words not recognized by individual students. Judy Montgomery (2007) indicates a sample of the various sources to find lists of words which are important for students to know. Robert

Marzano (2004) has also compiled lists of words across subject areas for students in grades K to 12. Research by Beck, Kucan, and McKoewan (2013) outlines the three tiers of vocabulary and demonstrates how to effectively choose Tier 2 words as a focus of explicit instruction.

One strategy for teaching word learning is to teach the student how to determine the meaning of unknown words using context and/or word parts. This skill is vital for a student to be able to move through the Common Core State Standards (CCSS), or specific state standards. In addition, students with language impairments often do not learn these strategies as typical learners do. Speech-language services in the school system should be reserved for students who require specialized instruction that would not be necessary for memorizing words and definitions. A student's IEP goals should not reflect the grade-level standard as that standard is taught in the classroom.

Prerequisite Skills	VOCABULARY Steps to Mastery of Skills/Goals

Nouns
Verbs
Pronouns
Adjectives
  Color
  Shape
  Size
  Function
  Sensory
  Number
Adverbs
	• Identify/name ___#___ _____ (nouns, verbs, etc.) from an object.
	• Identify/name ___#___ _____ (nouns, verbs, etc.) from a picture of a single item.
	• Name ___#___ items in a given category (household items, furniture, food, transportation, etc.).
	• Identify/name ___#___ _____ (nouns, verbs, etc.) from a picture scene or illustrated story.
	• Use _____ (nouns, verbs, etc.) in sentences.
	• Use _____ (nouns, verbs, etc.) in structured conversation.
	• Use _____ (nouns, verb, etc.) in unstructured conversation.

Match	• Match two objects when presented with ___#___ objects. • Match two pictures when presented with ___#___ pictures. • Point to pictures that are the same in a field of ___#___.
Sort	• Sort ___#___ objects when presented with ___#___ objects. • Sort ___#___ pictures when presented with ___#___ pictures.

Concepts
  Spatial
  Temporal
  Quantitative
  Qualitative
	• Identify/name *(state specific concepts) using objects.
	• Identify/name *(state specific concepts) using pictures.
	• Identify/name *(state specific concepts) using illustrated story.
	• Use *(state specific concepts) during academic instruction.
	*ex.: spatial, temporal, quantitative, qualitative.

Comparatives/ Superlatives	• Identify comparatives (big/bigger, small/smaller, etc.) when given two objects. • Identify comparatives when given two pictures of nouns. • Identify comparatives when given two pictures of verbs. • Identify comparatives when given a picture scene. • Identify superlatives (biggest, smallest, etc.) when given three objects. • Identify superlatives when given three pictures of nouns. • Identify superlatives when given three pictures of verbs. • Identify superlatives when given a picture scene. • Use comparatives and superlatives during academic instruction.

Prerequisite Skills	VOCABULARY Steps to Mastery of Skills/Goals
Categorize	• State ___#___ items when given a category. • State category when given ___#___ pictures/words. • Sort ___#___ pictures by attribute. • State shared attribute when given ___#___ pictures/words.
Negation	• Identify the item that represents "not" + noun from a choice of ___#___. • Identify the item that does not belong from a choice of ___#___.
Describe	• Describe object using ___#___ descriptors (state descriptors).* • Describe picture of a single item using ___#___ descriptors (state descriptors).* • Describe picture scene using ___#___ descriptors (state descriptors).* • Describe illustrated story using ___#___ descriptors.* • Describe situation using ___#___ descriptors.* *for example, action, adjective, concept, category, etc.
Compare/contrast	• State a similarity when given ___#___ pictures. • State ___#___ differences when given ___#___ pictures. • State ___#___ similarities and ___#___ differences when given two picture scenes. • State ___#___ similarities and ___#___ differences between ___#___ characters of a story. • State ___#___ similarities and ___#___ differences between two themes/topics/plots/stories.
Antonyms Synonyms	• State antonym of a given picture when given ___#___ choices. • State antonym of a given picture. • State antonym of a given word when given ___#___ choices. • State antonym of a given word. • State antonym of a given word within a sentence. • State antonym of a given word within a story. • State synonym of a given picture when given ___#___ choices. • State synonym of a given picture. • State synonym of a given word when given ___#___ choices. • State synonym of a given word. • State synonym of a given word within a sentence. • State synonym of a given word within a story. • State antonym and synonym of words during academic instruction.

Prerequisite Skills	VOCABULARY Steps to Mastery of Skills/Goals

Meaning from context
   Word parts
     Root
     Prefix
     Suffix
	• Answer yes/no questions about a sentence.
	• Answer yes/no questions about a paragraph.
	  (For yes/no questions, answer must be stated in sentence or paragraph.)
	• Answer factual questions about a sentence.
	• Answer factual questions about a paragraph.
	• Determine meaning of unknown words using context clues when given a choice of ___#___ definitions.
	• Identify information in text that supports meaning of unknown word.
	• State meaning of unknown word using context clues and use in a sentence that demonstrates the meaning.
	• Identify <u>(root, prefix, suffix)</u> of a word.
	• State meaning of root word.
	• State meaning of prefix <u>(state which prefixes)</u> of a word.
	• State meaning of suffix <u>(state which suffixes)</u> of a word.
	• State meaning of unknown word from word parts.
	• State meaning of unknown word using context clues and word parts and use in a sentence that demonstrates the meaning.

Multiple meaning words	• Point to a picture of a multiple meaning word when used in a sentence when given ___#___ pictures. • Point to pictures that represent meanings of a given word when given ___#___ pictures. • Use multiple meaning word in two different contexts that demonstrate understanding of the meanings.

QUESTIONS

The ability to ask and answer questions and demonstrate comprehension is essential for a student to proceed through the Early Learning Standards or access the Common Core State Standards and progress in the curriculum. This section breaks down the "wh-questions" into a hierarchy of development.

Speech-language pathologists (SLPs), spend a great deal of time addressing questions with students with language impairments. Once a student knows the difference between "telling" and "asking," the SLP should look at the continuum of question forms as it pertains to answering factual questions. This continuum begins with yes/no questions, which are followed by wh-questions. It is recommended that SLPs work on wh-questions in the following hierarchal order: *what, where, who, when, why, and how* (Bloom, Merkin, & Wootten, 1982; Rowland, Pine, Lieven, & Theaksston, 2003).

Asking yes/no questions can be an appropriate method of assessing comprehension or vocabulary development. When addressing yes/no questions in an IEP goal, the answer to the questions must always be known by the SLP in order for data collection to be accurate. For example, you might ask a student a vocabulary-related question, such as "Is this a ball?" or a comprehension-related question such as "Did the girl go to the store?" When utilizing yes/no questions, the answer to the question or request you present must be known by the SLP in order for data to be valid. For example, if a student is asked, "Do you want a cracker?" only the student would know if he or she wants a cracker. The SLP would not know if the student answered correctly.

Once the student has demonstrated that he or she can answer yes/no questions, move on to the wh-questions. Take into consideration the types of wh-questions a student is currently able to answer when developing IEP goals. A goal should not be as broad as to just state "wh-questions." It is more understandable and measureable if the goal specifically identifies which wh-questions (i.e., *what, where, who, when, why, how*) and whether the questions are factual or inferential. Also, the timeframe of the IEP must be taken into account. The SLP needs to determine what is reasonable for the student to attain by the mastery date. If a student is currently unable to answer "what" questions successfully, it may not be reasonable to expect them to answer "why" questions in the time frame of an IEP. When initially working on wh-questions, address factual questions first. An SLP should determine that a student can answer factual questions for all types of wh-question words before moving on to the next skill.

It is a common misconception that a *why* or *how* question is always an inferential question. In actuality, *why* and *how* questions can be factual or inferential. In addition, a *what, where, who,* or *when* question could require an inference. Let's consider some examples:

"She went to the store to buy milk. *Why* did she go to the store?" (factual)

"Jimmy fell and scraped his knee. *How* did he scrape his knee?" (factual)

"He found a ball light enough for him. He rolled it down the lane and knocked down eight pins. *Where* is he? "(inferential)

Prerequisite Skills	QUESTIONS Steps to Mastery of Skills/Goals
Knows difference between telling (declarative) and asking (interrogative)	• Identify a given sentence as a statement (declarative, exclamatory) or a question (interrogative).
Answer questions Yes/no What Where Who When Why How (Work on wh-questions in the above order)	• Answer factual yes/no questions about a picture. • Point to a picture that represents _____ (what, where, who, when, why, how) from a choice of ___#___. • Answer factual _____ (specify what, where, who, when, why, how) questions about a picture providing all required information. • Answer factual _____ (specify yes/no, what, where, who, when, why, how) questions about a picture scene providing all required information. • Answer factual _____ (specify yes/no, what, where, who, when, why, how) questions about a ___#___ sentence story providing all required information. • Answer factual _____ (specify yes/no, what, where, who, when, why, how) questions about a _____ (paragraph/short story/ situation) providing all required information. • Identify information in text to answer factual _____ (specify yes/no, what, where, who, when, why, how) questions.
Identify what information is needed	• Identify what you know in a picture. • Identify what's missing or what's wrong in a picture. • Identify what you know in a picture scene. • Identify what's missing or what's wrong in a picture scene. • Identify what you know in an instruction/question. • Identify what you want to know in an instruction/question. • Identify what you know in a (paragraph/story/text). • Identify what you want to know in a (paragraph/story/text). • Formulate a question based on what information is needed.
Narrative elements Characters Setting Events	• Answer factual questions about narrative elements (character, setting, events) from a _____ (paragraph/short story) providing all required information. • Answer factual questions about narrative elements (character, setting, events) from a _____ (chapter/story) providing all required information.

Prerequisite Skills	QUESTIONS Steps to Mastery of Skills/Goals
Cause/effect	• Identify effect when given a cause in a picture scene. • Identify effect when given a cause in a sentence. • Identify a cause when given an effect in a picture scene. • Identify a cause when given an effect in a sentence. • Answer cause and effect questions about a picture scene. • Answer cause and effect questions about a sentence. • Answer cause and effect questions about a paragraph/situation. • Answer cause and effect questions about a _____ (chapter/story).
Infer/draw conclusions	• Answer inferential questions about a _____ (picture scene or sentence) providing all required information. • Provide evidence from _____ (picture scene or sentence) and background knowledge to support an inference. • Answer inferential questions about a paragraph or situation providing all required information. • Provide evidence from a paragraph or situation and background knowledge to support an inference. • Answer inferential questions about narrative elements (characters, setting, events) from a _____ (chapter, story, etc.) providing all required information. • Provide evidence from a _____ (chapter, story, etc.) and background knowledge to support an inference.

SUMMARIZE

The skill of summarizing builds on the skills of sequencing and retelling. The *Summarize* section is broken down into the prerequisite skills that lead to each skill's development. There are subtle differences between the skills of retelling and summarizing. For the purposes of this book, the breakdown of the prerequisite skills and steps to mastery are based on the following descriptions of these similar skills. Both retelling and summarizing require that the information be put into a student's own words, or paraphrased. A retell can be explained as paraphrasing information in sequence using the basic narrative elements of characters, setting, and events. A summary is paraphrased information that is much shorter in length than the original and contains only the most important, main points (Conrad-Curry, 2013).

SLPs should be aware that the lowest-level prerequisite skills for this section overlap with the *Questions* section. There are also specific vocabulary concepts required for the skill of sequencing. If a student is not at the level of answering factual yes/no questions about a picture or is missing essential concepts, the SLP should consider returning to the *Questions* and/or *Vocabulary* sections for lower-level prerequisite skills.

Prerequisite Skills	SUMMARIZE Steps to Mastery of Skills/Goals

Answer questions
  Yes/no
  What
  Where
  Who
  When
  Why
  How
 	
(Work on
wh-questions in
the above order)
	• Answer factual _____ (specify yes/no, what, where, who, when, why, how) questions about a picture providing all required information.
	• Answer factual _____ (specify yes/no, what, where, who, when, why, how) questions about a picture scene providing all required information.
	• Answer factual _____ (specify yes/no, what, where, who, when, why, how) questions about a ___#___ sentence story providing all required information.
	• Answer factual _____ (specify yes/no, what, where, who, when, why, how) questions about a (paragraph/short story/situation) providing all required information.
	• Identify information in text to answer factual _____ (specify yes/no, what, where, who, when, why, how) questions.

Sequence concepts
  Beginning,
  middle, end,
  last, before/
  after, next
  Ordinals (1st,
  2nd, etc.)
  Yesterday,
  today,
  tomorrow
	• Identify ___*___ of a row/line.
	• Identify ___*___ of a ___#___ picture sequence.
	• Answer questions about a ___#___ picture sequence (related to sequence details).
	
	(*Beginning, middle, end, before, after, first, second, last, etc.)

Sequence	• Sequence ___#___ pictures. • Sequence ___#___ academic instructions.

Narrative elements
  Characters
  Setting
  Events
	• Answer factual questions about narrative elements (characters, setting, events) from a chapter/story/poem providing all required information.

Prerequisite Skills	SUMMARIZE Steps to Mastery of Skills/Goals
Retell	• Rephrase a picture description. • Rephrase academic instructions. • Retell routine/story of a ___#___ picture sequence. • Retell routine/personal experience/story in his/her own words (without picture support).
Important versus unimportant details	• Determine important from unimportant details in a picture scene. • Determine important from unimportant details in a ___#___ sentence story. • Determine important from unimportant details in a _____ (story/chapter, discussion, etc.).
Summarize	• Summarize ___#___ details from a _____ (short story, chapter, text, etc.).

MAIN IDEA AND DETAILS

The ability to identify main ideas and details is essential to comprehension of instruction and text (Byrne, 2005). There is a great deal of overlap in this *Main Idea and Details* section with the skills in the *Questions* and *Summarize* sections. If a student cannot successfully reach the lowest level for this skill area (e.g., answering factual questions), the SLP should go back to the *Questions* section for lower level prerequisite skills.

The skills of main idea and details also develop at varying levels. A student in the lower, elementary grades would be expected to identify the topic and then move toward identifying a stated main idea. Beginning prerequisite skills for *Main Idea* will also be found in the *Questions* and *Summarize* sections. Students in higher grades are expected to identify a main idea by inferring from the supporting details (Byrne, 2005). In this section, the final prerequisite skill a student is expected to master is the ability to infer the main idea and determine the supporting details.

Prerequisite Skills	MAIN IDEA AND DETAILS Steps to Mastery of Skills/Goals

Answer questions
    Yes/no
    What
    Where
    Who
    When
    Why
    How
 	
(Work on
wh-questions in
the above order)
	• Answer factual _____ (specify yes/no, what, where, who, when, why, how) questions about a picture providing all required information.
	• Answer factual _____ (specify yes/no, what, where, who, when, why, how) questions about a picture scene providing all required information.
	• Answer factual _____ (specify yes/no, what, where, who, when, why, how) questions about a ___#___ sentence story providing all required information.
	• Answer factual _____ (specify yes/no, what, where, who, when, why, how) questions about a _____ (paragraph/short story/situation) providing all required information.
	• Identify information in text to answer factual _____ (specify yes/no, what, where, who, when, why, how) questions.

Sequence
    Beginning,
    middle, end,
    last
    Before/after,
    next
    Ordinals (1st,
    2nd, etc.)
    Yesterday,
    today,
    tomorrow
	• Identify ___*___ of a row/line.
	• Identify ___*___ of a ___#___ picture sequence.
	• Answer questions about a ___#___ picture sequence (related to sequence details).
	(*Beginning, middle, end, before, after, first, second, last, etc.)
	• Sequence ___#___ pictures.
	• Sequence ___#___ academic instructions.

Main idea when stated	• Identify topic of paragraph/story. • Identify main idea when stated in the paragraph/story.
Important versus unimportant details	• Determine important from unimportant details in picture scene. • Determine important from unimportant details in a ___#___ sentence story. • Determine important from unimportant details in a _____ (story/chapter, discussion, etc.).

Prerequisite Skills	MAIN IDEA AND DETAILS Steps to Mastery of Skills/Goals
Infer/draw conclusions	• Identify a supporting detail when given a choice of three and given the main idea in a _____ (paragraph, story, poem, chapter, etc.). • Identify ___#___ details that support a given main idea in a _____ (paragraph, story, poem, chapter, etc.). • Identify ___#___ important details in a _____ (paragraph, story, poem, chapter, etc.) when the main idea is not known. • Identify main idea of a _____ (paragraph, story, poem, chapter, etc.) and provide ___#___ supporting details.

CRITICAL THINKING

The *Critical Thinking* area outlines the higher-level language skills, including cause and effect, predicting, and making inferences. Once a student is at the level of *Critical Thinking*, he or she is expected to have the skills from each of the previous areas, that is, *Vocabulary, Questions, Summarize,* and *Main Idea and Details.* Although there is an overlap of skills from these areas, it does not indicate the full list of prerequisite skills for each overlapping skill. For example, the prerequisite skill of 'Answer factual questions' is the lowest level prerequisite in the *Critical Thinking* area. However, this skill itself has other prerequisite skills as indicated in the *Questions* area. If the student is not ready for the *Steps to Mastery* for the prerequisite skills in the *Critical Thinking* area, the SLP should refer back to the respective area(s) for lower-level skills.

Prerequisite Skills	CRITICAL THINKING Steps to Mastery of Skills/Goals
Answer factual questions	• Answer factual questions about a _____ (paragraph/short story/ situation) providing all required information. • Identify information in text to answer factual questions.
Sequence	• Sequence ___#___ pictures. • Provide ___#___ details, in sequential order, of a _____ (story, chapter, situation, etc.).
Important versus unimportant details	• Determine important from unimportant details in a ___#___ sentence, story. • Determine important from unimportant details in a _____ (story/ chapter, discussion, etc.).
Compare/contrast	• State ___#___ similarities and ___#___ differences when given two picture scenes. • State ___#___ similarities and ___#___ differences between ___#___ characters of a story. • State ___#___ similarities and ___#___ differences between two _____ (themes/topics/plots/ stories).
Cause/effect	• Identify effect when given a cause about a picture scene or sentence. • Identify a cause when given an effect about a picture scene or sentence. • Answer cause and effect questions about a picture scene or sentence. • Answer cause and effect questions about a _____ (paragraph, situation, etc.). • Answer cause and effect questions about a _____ (chapter, story, etc.).
Predict	• Predict what will happen based on title and story cover and provide evidence for that prediction. • Predict what will happen next when provided with ___#___ pictures and provide evidence for that prediction. • Predict what will happen next in a situation/real life experience and provide evidence for that prediction. • Predict what will happen next in a _____ (story, chapter, etc.) and provide evidence for that prediction.

Prerequisite Skills	CRITICAL THINKING Steps to Mastery of Skills/Goals
Problem solve	• Identify the problem in a picture. • Identify the problem in a picture scene. • Identify the problem in a situation. • Identify the problem in a paragraph. • Identify the problem in a _____ (short story, chapter, etc.). • Brainstorm two possible solutions to a given problem. • Identify best solution for a given problem. • Explain why a solution was chosen for a given problem. • Identify problem and provide solution using grade level curriculum-based materials.
Infer/draw conclusions	• Answer inferential questions about a _____ (picture scene or sentence) providing all required information. • Provide evidence from _____ (picture scene or sentence) and background knowledge to support an inference. • Answer inferential questions about a paragraph or situation providing all required information. • Provide evidence from a paragraph or situation and background knowledge to support an inference. • Answer inferential questions about narrative elements (characters, setting, events) from a _____ (chapter, story, etc.) providing all required information. • Provide evidence from a _____ (chapter, story, etc.) and background knowledge to support an inference.
Nonliteral language Figurative language	• Provide literal interpretation of nonliteral statement. • Determine if literal interpretation makes sense. • Determine meaning of nonliteral statement using context. • Provide literal statement that demonstrates the meaning of a nonliteral statement.
Fact/opinion	• Explain what a fact is. • Explain what an opinion is. • Provide detail(s) to support a given fact. • Identify opinion when given a choice of three. • Explain why a given statement is an opinion. • Identify statements within a paragraph/story as fact or opinion.

PRAGMATICS

SLPs are often the first person sought out when a student is exhibiting social skill deficits. While the SLP alone should not be targeting all social skills, this individual can provide support and training related to pragmatics.

The hierarchy within the *Pragmatics* section is broken down in a slightly different way than earlier sections. Rather than being listed as "Prerequisite Skills," the first column is titled "Skills." This is because pragmatics, unlike areas discussed previously, develop in a much more simultaneous manner. Students with social-communication deficits are more likely to exhibit splinter skills. However, within each of the pragmatic skills, there is a hierarchy of *Steps to Mastery* needed to master that skill. For example, in order to master the use of greetings/farewells, a student must achieve the following skills:

- Nonverbal acknowledgment

- Body oriented toward person

- Face oriented toward person

- Produce greetings and farewells ("hi," "bye") when entering or leaving a room

Another aspect of pragmatics is that the majority of skills require an underlying level of language. With the exception of very basic pragmatic skills, such as "Greetings/Farewells" and "Request for Object or Action," social communication requires skills in all the previous sections. For example, drawing inferences occurs often in conversations and is an important skill for taking perspective.

The skill of eye contact is not specifically addressed in the *Pragmatics* section. There are different theories (some of which are contradictory) regarding the need for establishing eye contact in social situations. Often, when working on eye contact, people think that means constantly looking at the individual with whom you are communicating. In reality, and depending on age, the individual will glance at the person he or she is talking to, and then glance away. In addition, eye contact can make social interaction and conversations more difficult for students with social language deficits. When those students are thinking of what to say, they often need to look away to think about what they are saying (Stewart, n.d.; Winner, 2007). Students with pragmatic language deficits, including those with Autism Spectrum Disorders, may need to be explicitly taught such skills; such as, the purpose of using their eyes, following a gaze, establishing joint attention, and the Theory of Mind (Winner, 2007). *Steps to Mastery* address these skills and are included in the *Pragmatics* section.

Prerequisite Skills	PRAGMATICS Steps to Mastery of Skills/Goals
Greetings Farewells	• Nonverbal acknowldgement • Body oriented toward person • Face oriented toward person • Produce greetings and farewells (hi, bye) when entering or leaving a room.
Request for object or action	• Indicate (points to, verbalizes, reaches for, etc.) desire for _____ (object/action). • Label _____ (object/action). • Request desired _____ (object or action) using _____ (# words, whole sentence, etc.).
Identify own emotions	• Identify emotions through pictures, social stories, role playing, or video modeling. • State own emotion/feeling in a role-play situation or video modeling. • State own emotion/feeling when in a real-life situation.
Nonverbal cues	• Identify others' emotions through pictures, social stories, role playing or video modeling. • Identify different types of body language through pictures, social stories, role playing, or video modeling: ○ where eyes are looking ○ position of body ○ tone of voice ○ gestures ○ proximity ○ facial expression • Brainstorm meaning of others' nonverbal cues. • Respond to nonverbal cues by changing behavior, language, or nonverbal response.
Request help, information, clarification	• Identify what you know. • Identify when help/information/clarification is needed. • Request _____ (help, information, clarification) when needed.

Prerequisite Skills	PRAGMATICS Steps to Mastery of Skills/Goals
Responding	<ul><li>Acknowledge speaker:<ul><li>orient body toward speaker</li><li>orient face toward speaker</li></ul></li><li>Brainstorm ideas of how to respond.</li><li>Respond to speaker by _____ (pointing, verbalizing, etc.).</li></ul>
Protesting	<ul><li>Identify that he or she disagrees with the situation or what the person says.</li><li>Brainstorm different ways to express disagreement.</li><li>Determine the best way to disagree.</li><li>Appropriately (verbally or nonverbally) demonstrate disagreement.</li></ul>
Conversational repairs	<ul><li>Acknowledge the listener is not understanding:<ul><li>nonverbal cue</li><li>verbal cue</li></ul></li><li>Repair utterances when not understood by the listener.</li></ul>
Problem solve	<ul><li>Identify the problem in a picture.</li><li>Identify the problem in a picture scene.</li><li>Identify the problem in a situation/social story.</li><li>Brainstorm two possible solutions.</li><li>Determine the best solution.</li><li>Explain why the solution was chosen.</li><li>Identify problem and the solution in a real-life situation.</li></ul>
Taking perspective of others	<ul><li>Identify that others can have a different viewpoint/attitude/idea.</li><li>Explain two viewpoints/ideas for a given topic/situation.</li><li>Identify viewpoints/attitudes/ideas of characters in a _____ paragraph/ story/chapter/situation.</li><li>Identify when conversational partner has a different viewpoint/attitude/idea.</li><li>Accept other person's perspective:<ul><li>not arguing</li><li>not insisting</li></ul></li></ul>

Prerequisite Skills	PRAGMATICS Steps to Mastery of Skills/Goals
Initiating conversation	• Determine if it is a good time to talk to the person. • Choose an appropriate topic for setting/situation. • Orient face and body to the listener. • Initiate conversation with listening partner(s).
Topic maintenance, joining in Exiting Ending	• Identify topic/main idea of conversation. • Brainstorm ideas to respond to the topic. • Identify when to add to the topic. • Respond to speaker maintaining same/related topic for ___#___ turns. • Identify what to say when leaving or ending a conversation in role playing situations. • Identify what to say when leaving or ending a conversation in real-life situations.
Nonliteral language Figurative language	• Identify nonliteral statement/sentence. • Provide literal interpretation of nonliteral statement. • Determine if the literal interpretation makes sense. • Determine meaning of nonliteral statement using context. • Provide literal statement that demonstrates the meaning of a nonliteral statement.

SYNTAX AND MORPHOLOGY

The prerequisite skills within the *Syntax and Morphology* section have been arranged according to developmental acquisition; however skills often develop simultaneously. As there are many resources that address the development of syntax and morphology skills, the representative research of several authors was selected (Dawson, Stout, & Eyer, 2003; Gard, Gilman, & Gorman, 1993; Morris, n.d.). The *Syntax and Morphology* section takes into account that students have basic skills of vocabulary and concepts. These include a range of nouns and verbs, concept of more than one, and spatial concepts. Each syntax and morphology skill is broken down into the prerequisite skills needed for mastery. For example, in order to master the skills of present progressives, a student would be expected to have the following skills:

- Verbs

- Singular versus plural

- Present participle (ing)

- Helping "to be" verbs (Is/Am/Are)

Knowing that a student has the above prerequisite skills in place, the SLP can then better develop a goal using the *Steps to Mastery of Skills* for present progressive:

- Use "am," "is," "are," and "ing":
  - in a phrase
  - in a sentence
  - in structured conversation
  - in unstructured conversation
  - during academic instruction

When considering the need for goals that address syntax and morphology, an SLP should also take into account the Early Learning Standards, the Common Core State Standards (CCSS), or specific state standards. Also considered should be the age/grade level the students are expected to be consistent with the skill. For example, irregular plurals for commonly occurring nouns should be consistent by age 5;0 (Dawson et al., 2003; Gard et al., 1993). However, the CCSS for Language indicates 2nd graders should *"Form and use frequently occurring irregular plural nouns (e.g., feet, children, teeth, mice, fish)"* (NGA & CCSSO, 2010). Irregular, past tense verbs are often consistent at 4 years of age; however, the CCSS has this skill at 2nd grade: *"Form and use the past tense of frequently occurring irregular verbs (e.g., sat, hid, told)"* (Dawson et al., 2003; Gard et al., 1993; NGA & CCSSO, 2010). Therefore, one should not solely use developmental norms, but also use the state standards as a guide. If a skill is addressed in the state standards and is part of the curriculum during that school year, it should not be written as an IEP goal.

Prerequisite Skills	SYNTAX AND MORPHOLOGY Steps to Mastery of Skills/Goals

Sentence construction
 	
Subject
Object
Verb
	• Use ___*___ during _____ (structured conversation or unstructured conversation):
	    * subject + object (Boy book)
	    * subject + verb (Cat ran)
	    * subject + verb + object (Boy read book)

Articles (the, a, an)
 	
Prepositional phrases
 	
Conjunctions (and, but, because)
	• Use _____ (specify prepositional phrase, article and/or conjunction):
	  ○ in a phrase
	  ○ in a sentence
	  ○ in structured conversation
	  ○ in unstructured conversation
	  ○ during academic instruction

Present progressive
 	
Verbs
 	
Singular versus plural
 	
Present participle (ing)
 	
Helping "to be" verbs (is/am/are)
	• Point to a picture that represents "is" or "are" + verbing from a choice of ___#___.
	• Use "am," "is," "are," and "ing":
	  ○ in a phrase
	  ○ in a sentence
	  ○ in structured conversation
	  ○ in unstructured conversation
	  ○ during academic instruction

Plurals Singular versus plural More than one Regular "s" "es" Irregular (commonly occurring)	• Identify if noun refers to one or more than one • Identify _____ (regular or irregular) plural of a given noun from a choice of ___#___ • Use _____ (regular or irregular) plurals in a sentence • Use _____ (regular or irregular) plurals in structured conversation • Use _____ (regular or irregular) plurals in unstructured conversation • Use _____ (regular or irregular) plurals during academic instruction

Prerequisite Skills	SYNTAX AND MORPHOLOGY Steps to Mastery of Skills/Goals

Past tense
 	
Present tense versus past tense
 	
"ed" = past
 	
Regular past tense
 	
Irregular past tense
	• Use (regular or irregular) past tense:
	  ◦ in phrases
	  ◦ in sentences
	  ◦ in structured conversation
	  ◦ in unstructured conversation
	  ◦ during academic instruction

Pronouns
 	
Singular versus plural
 	
Subject of a sentence
 	
Object of a sentence
 	
Possessives
	• Point to the picture that represents a given pronoun from a choice of ___#___.
	• State pronoun for a given picture.
	• Use pronouns:
	  ◦ in phrases
	  ◦ in sentences
	  ◦ in structured conversation
	  ◦ in unstructured conversation
	  ◦ during academic instruction

Possessives
 	
Concept of ownership (belong to)
 	
Addition of s/z sound
	• Point to the picture that shows possession from a choice of ___#___.
	• Use possessives:
	  ◦ in words
	  ◦ in sentences
	  ◦ in structured conversation
	  ◦ in unstructured conversation
	  ◦ during academic instruction

Present tense
 	
Singular versus plural
 	
Present tense versus past tense
 	
Third person singular "s"
	• Use present tense:
	  ◦ in phrases
	  ◦ in sentences
	  ◦ in structured conversation
	  ◦ in unstructured conversation
	  ◦ during academic instruction

Prerequisite Skills	SYNTAX AND MORPHOLOGY Steps to Mastery of Skills/Goals

Future tense
 	
Present tense versus past tense versus future tense
 	
Will + verb
 	
Am/is/are + going to + verb
 	
Will be + verb "ing"
 	
Am/is/are + going to be + verb + ing
	• Use future tense:
	  ◦ in words
	  ◦ in sentences
	  ◦ in structured conversation
	  ◦ in unstructured conversation
	  ◦ during academic instruction

Comparatives/ superlatives
 	
Adjectives
 	
Concept of "comparisons" "-er" "-est"
 	
Irregular adjectives (good, better, best)
	• Point to the picture that represents adjective + "er" from a choice of two.
	• Use comparatives:
	  ◦ in words
	  ◦ in sentences
	  ◦ in structured conversation
	  ◦ in unstructured conversation
	  ◦ during academic instruction
	• Point to the picture that represents adjective + "est" from a choice of three.
	• Use comparatives and superlatives:
	  ◦ in words
	  ◦ in sentences
	  ◦ in structured conversation
	  ◦ in unstructured conversation
	  ◦ during academic instruction

ARTICULATION AND PHONOLOGICAL PROCESSES °

The *Articulation and Phonological Processes* section separates out the developmental norms for articulation sounds and phonological processes. The developmental age listed for articulation is the age in which 90% of children have mastered the sound based on an average of multiple resources (Goldman & Fristoe, 2000; Sander, 1972; Smit, Hand, Freilinger, Bernthal, & Bird, 1990). The age at which a phonological process is expected to be extinguished is also based on an average from various resources; all processes should be extinguished by age five (Bowen, 2012; Hodson, 2011). This book includes the most common phonological processes.

The hierarchy of sound production is indicated from discrimination to unstructured conversation. However, discrimination is not indicated under *Steps to Mastery* for IEP goal development. Discrimination may be the entry point of intervention for a given student, but the goal would be developed for production of a specific sound, even if in isolation with lower criteria for mastery.

Parents and teachers are important, active members of the IEP team. As such, it is imperative that IEP goals include terminology that both parents and teachers can easily understand. Many of the SLP terms are unfamiliar to these team members. Phonological processes is one of these areas. IEP goals in this area are often written to reduce the occurrence of a specific phonological process. For example, "The student will reduce the process of fronting." Whereas many SLPs are trained to use this framework, it can be difficult to write these goals in a clear, measureable way.

In this book, the Phonological Processes *Steps to Mastery* are specifically written to represent what the student is expected to produce, rather than as the extinguishing of the phonological process the student displays. For example, instead of writing a goal to "reduce the phonological process of final consonant deletion in words," the goal could be developed as "produce final consonants in words." This helps keep the goal understandable, doable, and measureable while using parent-friendly terminology. If an individual SLP or school district feels there is a need to mention the specific phonological process in the goal, there are still ways to do this within our proposed model. For example, a goal could be written as, "To reduce cluster reduction, student will produce two sounds for each blend" or "Student will produce the back sounds of /k/ and /g/ to reduce the process of fronting." Regardless of whether one is treating single sound articulation errors, one phonological process, or multiple phonological processes, the IEP goals can be developed utilizing the *Steps to Mastery* presented in this section.

When developing goals for articulation or phonological processes, it is important to consider what level of production—from isolation to unstructured conversation—the student can achieve in the timeframe of the IEP. An IEP does not need to include goals for each step. Let us consider a student who is currently producing /l/ at the word level with 80% accuracy in 4/5 trials. While the next step in the hierarchy is for production at the sentence level, the SLP may recommend the next IEP goal at the structured conversation level due to the student's history of progress and carryover with the skill. On the other hand, it may not be reasonable for a student at the isolation level to move all the way to the structured conversation level in the course of one IEP.

With students who are highly unintelligible, the focus would be on increasing intelligibility as opposed to specific sounds or processes. For example, when utilizing the "Cycles" approach, the therapy concentrates on the emergence of specific sounds or patterns, rather than mastery (Bowen, n.d.). Therefore, a goal to improve overall intelligibility would be better than targeting the process(es) or sound(s); for example, "The student will increase intelligibility to 60% as measured by a familiar listener."

The goals for articulation and phonological processes may also focus on approximation of error sounds. This would especially be true for lower functioning students with significantly decreased intelligibility or for developmental errors when educational impact is documented. Educational impact for articulation should take both academic and social performance into consideration. Social performance can include intelligibility, class participation and teasing. This impact should be clearly documented.

Articulation

There must be a documented educational impact (academic or social).

Age	Skill	Steps to Mastery of Skills/Goals	
3	/b, p, m, n, h, w/	• Produce _____ (specify sounds) in _____	Discrimination Isolation
4	/k, g, d, f, j, t/		Syllables Words
6	/r, l/		Sentences
7	/tʃ, ʃ, dʒ, θ, ð, ŋ, v/		Structured conversation
8	*/s, z, ʒ/		Unstructured conversation
	*Developmental age does not apply to lateralization.		
	Intelligibility	• Increase intelligibility to _____% with unfamiliar listeners.**	
	**This applies to students for whom overall intelligibility is being targeted.		

Phonological Processes

There must be a documented educational impact (academic or social).

Age	Skill	Steps to Mastery of Skills/Goals	
3;3	final consonant deletion /boʊt/=/boʊ/	• Produce final consonant in _____	Discrimination Isolation (does not apply for final consonant deletion or weak syllable deletion) Words Sentences Structured conversation Unstructured conversation
3;6	velar fronting /kæp/=/tæp/	• Produce /k, g/ in _____	
4;0	weak syllable deletion /tɛləfon/=/tɛfon/	• Produce all syllables in 3-syllable words in _____	
4;0	cluster reduction /stɑr/=/tɑr/	• Produce 2 sounds for each blend in _____	
5;0	gliding of liquids*	• Produce close approximation of /l/ and /r/ in _____	
*The liquid consonants /l/ and /r/ are replaced by /w/ or /j/. /riəl/=/wiəl/; /lɪk/=/jɪk/ or /wɪk/; NOT /mʌðər/=/mʌðə/			
3;0	stopping /f, s/ /fud/=/tud/; /sɑk/=/dɑk/	• Produce _____ (specify sounds) in _____	
3;6	stopping /v, z/ /vɛri/=/bɛri/; /zu/=/du/		
4;6	stopping sh, j, ch /ʃu/=/du/; /dʒækət/=/dækət/; /tʃɑp/=/tɑp/		
5;0	stopping th /θʌm/=/tʌm/; /ðoz/=/doz/		

4

Writing IEP Goals

Writing Individualized Education Plan (IEP) goals can be the most difficult part of the IEP. A well written goal must describe the student's expected outcome within a given time. The goals need to be reflected in the present levels of the IEP. There are various frameworks for writing IEP goals, most notably SMART goals, which describes IEP goals as being Specific, Measurable, using Action words, Realistic and Relevant, and Time-limited (Wright & Wright, 2006).

In this book, this framework is described using four key words to remember when writing IEP goals:

- Understandable

- Doable

- Measureable

- Achievable

Goals should be *understandable* so that anyone reading them is able to understand what is being measured. This refers to the "**S**—Specific" and "**A**—uses Action words" of the SMART goals. When broadly interpreted words, such as "identify" or "determine" are used, they may cause confusion as to what exactly is being measured. How the student is expected to "identify" or "determine" must be specified; words such as "state" or "point to" are much clearer. The key word *"doable"* means that the goal must be at an appropriate level for the student, and all the prerequisite skills connected to it must be able to be executed. This easily corresponds with "**R**—Realistic and Relevant" goals. The *measureable* key word means that the goal targeted must be able to be measured. The key word *"achievable"* is interpreted such that it needs to be a "**R**—Realistic" expectation of what the student should be able to achieve in the course of the "**T**—Time-limited" IEP.

Regardless of which terminology or framework an SLP, state or school system utilizes, all IEP goals should incorporate the following ideas:

- The goals are based on the areas of needs that have been identified in the present level of performance in the IEP.

- The goals reflect where the student is expected to be by the end of the IEP or mastery date.

- The goals are aligned with state standards.

- The goals are skill-based.

- The goals are specific as to what you want the student to do and how you want the student to perform the task.

- The goals reflect the levels of support the student will receive (e.g. prompts or cues), if appropriate.

The goals should incorporate the mandates of the Federal Government's Individuals with Disabilities Education Act of 2004 (IDEA). This act states the following is required in the IEP:

(2)(i) A statement of measurable annual goals, including academic and functional goals designed to—

(A) Meet the child's needs that result from the child's disability to enable the child to be involved in and make progress in the general education curriculum; and

(B) Meet each of the child's other educational needs that result from the child's disability . . . [§300.320(a)(2)(i)(A) and (B)]

IDEA 2004 further states that an IEP must contain:

(3) A description of—

(i) How the child's progress toward meeting the annual goals described in paragraph (2) of this section will be measured; and

(ii) When periodic reports on the progress the child is making toward meeting the annual goals (such as through the use of quarterly or other periodic reports, concurrent with the issuance of reports cards) will be provided . . . [§300.320(a)(3)]

With the passing of IDEA 2004, benchmarks (intermediary steps toward meeting the goal) or short-term objectives (parallel tasks that support meeting the goal) are no longer required, except for a student who takes alternate assessments aligned to alternate achievement standards [§300.320(a)(2)(ii))] (U.S. Department of Education, 2004). Some school systems may require benchmarks or short-term objectives for all students. Since the law states that only annual goals are required in the IEP for the majority of disabled students, this book specifically addresses annual goals. For benchmarks or short-term objectives, the annual goal can easily be broken down into smaller steps by using the *Steps to Mastery*. Also, level of cues or prompting can be delineated in the benchmarks to show movement from maximum support to minimum or no support.

Goals written prior to an IEP meeting are considered a draft. The final result needs to be achieved by the entire IEP team (minimally, the SLP, the classroom teacher(s), and parent(s)) working together. Also, prior to an IEP meeting, it is imperative that the involved special education teachers collaborate in the drafting of the goals. A student should not have duplicate goals, that is, one written by the SLP, and a similar one written by the special education teacher. The same skill may be addressed by the special education teacher and the SLP, but the goal does not need to be written by both service providers in the IEP. If the student is working at a level that can be addressed adequately from the instruction of the teacher, then the student may not need additional specialized instruction from the SLP on that skill.

Although there are four areas of language—listening, speaking, reading, and writing — this book focuses on listening and speaking. When working with a student on comprehension, the SLP must be careful to separate out *reading* comprehension from *listening* comprehension. Even if the student is given a copy of a passage to follow along while text is read aloud, listening comprehension should be the focus of the student's goal.

Consider the following examples of reading versus listening goals. "The student will state the main idea and three supporting details after a short story has been read." This goal implies that the student will be reading the short story in which case reading comprehension is the focus. Also, a grade level has not been specified. The ultimate target would be to have the student achieve this goal at grade level. If the goal is written as "The student will identify the main idea and three supporting details after a grade-level short story has been read to him or her," then listening comprehension is the focus and a grade-level expectancy has been specified. However, if a 6th grade student is currently functioning at the 3rd grade level, it might not be realistic to expect the student to be performing on grade level for that skill by the end of the IEP. An example of a goal for this student would be, "The student will identify the main idea and three supporting details after a story has been read to him or her at their instructional level."

When writing goals, avoid using words that are either non-measureable or could cause confusion about what should be measured.

Measurable		Not Measureable	
Point	Draw	Improve	Feel
State	Describe	Practice	Explore
Complete	Answer	Know	Determine
Write	Sequence	Appropriate	Demonstrate understanding
		Identify	

The role of the SLP is to support the standards, not directly teach them. Therefore, when writing annual goals, the SLP must refer to the state standards. To review the process discussed in the preface, the SLP needs to determine what prerequisite speech-language skills are necessary to progress with a student's grade-level standards. The SLP would then look up the prerequisite speech-language skills in Chapter 3. Each *Prerequisite Skill* has a correlated list of *Steps to Mastery*. The SLP should determine where the student is currently functioning and what is realistic in terms of expected progress. The timeframe of the IEP should also be considered when determining what *Prerequisite Skills* and corresponding *Steps to Mastery* to target. Most IEPs are written for one year. The SLP should recommend what goals the student can reasonably achieve in the course of the IEP.

When developing goals, <u>all</u> the *Prerequisite Skills* and corresponding *Steps to Mastery* need to be considered. However, when writing the goals for the student's IEP, a goal is not written for each step to mastery; the goal is written for the prerequisite speech-language skills that need to be targeted.

Here are the steps to determine which *Prerequisite Skills* and corresponding *Steps to Mastery* should be targeted.

First:	Identify the grade-level state standards that coincide with the areas of difficulty.

Then:	Determine which prerequisite speech-language skills the student is lacking or struggling with.

Then:	Determine the *Step to Mastery* where the student is currently functioning.

Finally:	Determine which *Step to Mastery* the student can reasonably achieve during the course of the IEP.

Example: A 4th grade student is having difficulty with reading/language arts.

First:	**Identify the grade-level standards that coincide with the area(s) of difficulty:** 4th Grade Reading-Informational Common Core State Standards (NGA & CCSSO, 2010)

Then:	**Determine which prerequisite speech-language skills the student is lacking or struggling with:** Compare/contrast, summarize

Then:	**Determine where, in the *Steps to Mastery*, the student is <u>currently</u> functioning:** Compare/contrast: Describe a situation using four descriptors Summarize: Determine important from unimportant details in a picture scene

Finally:	**Determine which *Steps to Mastery* the student can reasonably <u>achieve</u> during the course of the IEP:** Compare/contrast: State two similarities and two differences between two characters in a story Summarize: Summarize eight details from a short story

Each *Step to Mastery* does not need to be written as a goal. The goal is the end result of where you want the student to be at the end of the IEP.

WHAT TO INCLUDE IN A GOAL

When writing a goal, the following should be included:

- the skill to be worked on

- how the student is expected to respond

- what material will be used

- how the material will be presented

- cues/prompts/supports (if needed)

- how the skill will be measured

- the criteria for mastery

Different school systems might have different requirements for goal development and writing. The specific emphasis here is based on IDEA 2004 Federal Rules and Regulations and what is required to make a goal understandable and measurable (U.S. Department of Education, 2004).

The types and amounts of cues/prompts/supports will be highly dependent on several factors for each student. These include the student's current level of functioning, the co-existing disabilities/areas of eligibility, and the amount of *Prerequisite Skills* and *Steps to Mastery* requiring interventions. The student's goal is to be as independent as possible with the skills.

An example using the same 4th grade student above:

The level the student can achieve during the course of the IEP:

State two similarities and two differences between two characters of a story.

The skill to be worked on	Compare/contrast characters
How the student is expected to respond	Will state two similarities and two differences
What material will be used	Grade-level material
How material will be presented	Orally (out loud)
Cues/Prompts/Supports	Graphic organizer
How the skill will be measured	Data collection and work samples
Criteria for mastery	Three out of four opportunities

The final goal could be:

Using a graphic organizer, the student will state two similarities and two differences between two characters of a grade-level story read aloud to him in three out of four opportunities.

How the skill will be measured: data collection and work samples.

Addressing the second prerequisite skill of summarize:

The level the student can achieve during the course of the IEP:

Summarize eight details from a short story

The skill to be worked on	Summarize eight details
How the student is expected to respond	Orally
What material will be used	Grade level short story
How material will be presented	Read aloud to student
Cues/Prompts/Supports	Picture cues from story
How the skill will be measured	Data collection
Criteria for mastery	Four out of five opportunities

The final goal could be:

Using picture cues from a story, the student will summarize eight details from a grade-level short story that has been read to him or her in four out of five opportunities.

How the skill will be measured: data collection

The *Goal Writing Worksheet*, a reproducible worksheet for writing goals, can be found at the end of this chapter in Appendix 4–1.

When writing goals, it is important to state exactly what is being measured. Words such as "no more than," "at least," or ranges such as "1 to 3" should not be used. For example, "The student will state 8 to 10 items in a category." What would be considered mastery; 8 items, 9 items, or 10 items? A more measureable goal would be "The student will state 10 items when provided a category." This example is very clear as to what is being measured, should be understandable by anyone reading it, and is doable in that it can be addressed. It is achievable if it is a realistic expectation for the student. Also, when writing goals, if the student is expected to master the goal with cues, the type and amount of cueing must be specified. For example, "The student will state 10 items when provided a category with 1 verbal cue." If no cues/prompts/supports are written into the goal, mastery requires the student to perform the skill independently. Goals should not be exactly the same year after year. If a skill was not mastered and needs continued work, consider how the goal was written. Perhaps more supports, such as cues, are needed for the student to reach mastery. Goals should not be wordy. The goal should be concise and indicate what the student is expected to do. Goals should also be written with parent-friendly language, layman's terms. Some parents might not be familiar with words such as phonological process, syntax, and many of the other professional terms SLPs have been taught.

CRITERIA FOR MASTERY

Besides considering what is realistic for the student to master in the timeframe of the IEP, the criteria must also make sense. Too often SLPs write blanket criteria for mastery such as 70% proficiency. That means if the student achieves 70% proficiency one time he or she has met the criteria for mastery. It would be more appropriate to write 70% proficiency for three sessions. If the student achieved 70% three separate times, the goal will have been mastered. Another way to write this could be 70% proficiency in four out of five opportunities.

Example: The goal is targeting production of /k/ in all positions of a word with 70% proficiency in four out of five opportunities

Day 1/Opportunity 1: student receives 60% accuracy (6/10 responses correct)

Day 2/Opportunity 2: student receives 70% accuracy (7/10 responses correct)

Day 3/Opportunity 3: student receives 70% accuracy (7/10 responses correct)

Day 4/Opportunity 4: student receives 80% accuracy (8/10 responses correct)

Day 5/Opportunity 5: student receives 80% accuracy (8/10 responses correct)

Based on the above data, the student has met mastery by demonstrating 70% proficiency in four out of five opportunities.

When deciding the criteria for mastery, keep in mind four out of five is not always the same as 80% when measuring certain skills. There are times that a percentage for criteria does not make sense. The SLP may need to consider the number of opportunities a student will have to exhibit the skill in a data collection session. An example might be with the skill main idea. How many opportunities are there for a student to determine the main idea of a chapter during a therapy session? Consider the amount of time it will take to read each chapter and that each chapter has one main idea. In this situation, it might make more sense to write mastery in terms of opportunities such as four out of five opportunities. Opportunities can occur on different days.

MEASURING PROGRESS

Goals should be measured by all professionals who work with the student (i.e., SLP, classroom teacher(s), and any other service providers). If data collection is the method of evaluation for a goal, it does not imply that only the SLP collects the data. Additionally, the SLP should be observing the student's skills outside of the therapy room to determine generalization of a skill. A language sample can be used as data. Other tools, such as documented classroom teacher observations, checklists (Table 4–1), work samples, and data sheets, are invaluable pieces of information to evaluate a student's abilities. It is important to gather valuable information, but important as well to be cognizant of the amount of work staff and teachers have to complete on a daily basis for a multitude of students. While yes/no responses from a teacher (as in Table 4–1) may appear to be simplistic, the specificity is respectful of individuals' time restraints. The purpose of the performance update is to determine if the skills being addressed by the SLP are being generalized into the classroom.

When documenting progress in the IEP, it is appropriate to report where the student is performing on the *Prerequisite Skills* and corresponding *Steps to Mastery*. For example, the goal (ending point) may be addressing the skill of retelling a story without picture support, but the student is working on the prerequisite skill of retelling a short story in a three-picture sequence. The data for the prerequisite skill (retelling a three-picture short story) should be reported. However, the SLP may also want to do a data probe for the ending point (retelling a story without picture support) and report that data.

If minimal or no progress is being made on a goal, it is essential to look at the prerequisite skills for that goal. If a goal is not being mastered, it is possible the goal was written at too high a level for the student, or that interventions did not start at a low enough level for the student to be successful. There are some areas of deficit that a student may never be able to fully achieve. For those areas, the SLP can use strategies that will help the student strengthen that skill.

In this book some areas overlap, therefore the same *Prerequisite Skills* and *Steps to Mastery* may be written in more than one area. Some examples are in the areas of *Vocabulary* and *Summarize* or *Main Idea and Details* and *Critical Thinking*. The reason for this overlap is because many language skills require the same prerequisite skills.

Table 4–1. Performance Update

Performance Update		
Student: _____ Date: _____ Teacher: _____		
Goals: • Comprehends/answers "who" questions • Comprehends and/or uses basic concepts • Correctly say /f/ and /l/ sounds in conversation		
Who Questions Does the student:	Yes	No
• Demonstrate understanding of "who" questions		
• Answer "who" questions		

Basic Concepts
 Does the student:
 	
 • Demonstrate understanding of concepts expected of a 2nd grader
     ○ If no, what concepts are not mastered?
     _____		

• Verbally use concepts expected of a 2nd grader		
F & L Sounds Does the student: • Say the /f/ and /l/ sounds correctly when reading		
• Say the /f/ and /l/ sounds correctly when talking		
Comments:		
Overall Classroom Performance:		

When utilizing this book to develop goals, the words in parentheses are options to consider. The following example is from *Vocabulary*:

"Identify/name ___#___ _____ (noun, verbs, etc.) from a (picture scene or illustrated story)." This could be written as "Point to <u>five</u> <u>nouns</u> from a picture scene" or "Name <u>five</u> <u>verbs</u> from a picture scene." It could also be written as, "Name <u>three</u> <u>adjectives</u> from an illustrated story." The term "etc." should not be written in the goal as its meaning can be broadly interpreted.

It is important to remember the following tips. Goals should not be the *starting* point. The goals on an IEP are *endpoint*s, indicating where the student is expected to end up by the mastery date. The process is to work through the *Steps to Mastery* to reach the goal. Optimally, written goals should be understandable, doable, measureable, and achievable.

GOAL EXAMPLES

Steps to Mastery

Any of the *Steps to Mastery* for vocabulary can be developed into IEP goals. The SLP needs to determine which step would be an entry point for the student and which step would be an ending point. The entry point is the step where the student is currently functioning. This is where intervention should begin. The goal(s) placed in an IEP should represent the endpoint—what the student can reasonably attain in the IEP's timeframe. The student must then work through the *Steps to Mastery* to reach the goal. Use the following tips to help you transform the *Steps to Mastery* into goals.

- Use the *Goal Writing Worksheet* in Appendix 4–1.

- Replace a # sign with a number.

- Consider the options in parentheses when filling in the blanks.

- Replace the words *identify* or *determine* with a specific instruction that is measurable (e.g., point to, write, name, state).

- Remember that goals must be understandable, doable, measureable, and achievable.

Prerequisite Skills

Every skill has several prerequisite skills that must be mastered prior to mastery of the larger skill. Prerequisite skills are not aligned with specific age or grade level. Students at any age or grade level could have or lack any of these skills. The prerequisite skills are generally listed in a hierarchy; however, some develop simultaneously with differing degrees of difficulty. A student does not have to master every prerequisite skill before moving on to another area.

Vocabulary

Example 1

Prerequisite Skill: Concepts-Spatial

Step to Mastery: Identify/name *(state specific concepts) using objects

The skill to be worked on:	Spatial concepts (in, on, out, under, over)
How the student is expected to respond:	Physically manipulate
What material will be used:	Objects
How material will be presented:	Student asked to demonstrate concept with given objects
Cues/Prompts/Supports:	None
Criteria for mastery:	80% accuracy for three sessions
Final Goal: How the skill will be measured:	The student will physically manipulate objects to demonstrate the spatial concepts *in, on, out, under,* and *over* with 80% accuracy for three sessions. Data collection

Example 2

Prerequisite Skill: Nouns

Step to Mastery: Identify/name ___#___ (noun, verb, etc.) from a picture of a single item

The skill to be worked on:	Labeling food/snack items
How the student is expected to respond:	Will state/label
What material will be used:	Picture cards
How material will be presented:	Picture cards shown to the student
Cues/Prompts/Supports:	One verbal prompt
Criteria for mastery:	80% accuracy in four out of five opportunities
Final Goal: How the skill will be measured:	The student will state 10 food/snack items when presented with picture cards and given one verbal prompt with 80% accuracy in four out of five opportunities. Data collection

Example 3

Prerequisite Skill: Match

Step to Mastery: Point to pictures that are the same in a field of ___#___

The skill to be worked on:	Matching
How the student is expected to respond:	Point
What material will be used:	Pictures
How material will be presented:	Three pictures shown at the same time
Cues/Prompts/Supports:	None
Criteria for mastery:	80% accuracy for three sessions
Final Goal: How the skill will be measured:	The student will point to pictures that are the same in a field of three with 80% accuracy for three sessions. Data collection

Example 4

Prerequisite Skill: Meaning from Context

Step to Mastery: State meaning of unknown word using context clues and use in a sentence that demonstrates the meaning

The skill to be worked on:	Meaning of unknown words from context
How the student is expected to respond:	Will state
What material will be used:	Grade level text
How material will be presented:	Read aloud to student
Cues/Prompts/Supports:	One verbal prompt
Criteria for mastery:	70% accuracy in three out of four sessions
Final Goal:	The student will state the meaning of unknown words using context clues from grade-level text that has been read to him and use it in a sentence that demonstrates the meaning with 70% accuracy in three out of four sessions.
How the skill will be measured:	Data collection, work samples

Questions

Example 5

Prerequisite Skill: Answer what and where

Step to Mastery: Answer factual (specify yes/no, what, where, who, when, why, how) questions about a _____ (paragraph/short story/situation) providing all required information

The skill to be worked on:	What and where
How the student is expected to respond:	Will state
What material will be used:	Three paragraph grade level story
How material will be presented:	Read aloud to student
Cues/Prompts/Supports:	None
Criteria for mastery:	80% accuracy in three out of four sessions
Final Goal:	The student will answer *what* and *where* questions about a three paragraph grade level story that has been read to him and will provide all required information with 80% accuracy in three out of four sessions.
How the skill will be measured:	Data collection

Example 6

Prerequisite Skill: Infer/Draw conclusions

Step to Mastery: Answer inferential questions about a paragraph/situation providing all required information

The skill to be worked on:	Inferential questions
How the student is expected to respond:	Will state
What material will be used:	Grade level material or a situation
How paragraph will be presented:	Read aloud to the student
Cues/Prompts/Supports:	None
Criteria for mastery:	80% accuracy in three out of four opportunities
Final Goal:	After listening to a situation or grade-level paragraph, the student will answer inferential questions and will provide all required information with 80% accuracy in three out of four opportunities.
How the skill will be measured:	Data collection, work samples

Summarize

Example 7

Prerequisite Skill: Sequence

Step to Mastery: Sequence ___#___ pictures

The skill to be worked on:	Sequencing
How the student is expected to respond:	Put pictures in order
What material will be used:	Sequence story pictures
How material will be presented:	Pictures given to student
Cues/Prompts/Supports:	None
Criteria for mastery:	80% accuracy for four sessions
Final Goal: How the skill will be measured:	The student will sequence six pictures with 80% accuracy for four sessions. Data collection

Example 8

Prerequisite Skill: Retell

Step to Mastery: Retell routine/personal experience/story in his/her own words (without picture support)

The skill to be worked on:	Retell to include beginning, middle, and end
How the student is expected to respond:	Will state
What material will be used:	Grade level short story
How material will be presented:	Read aloud to student
Cues/Prompts/Supports:	None
Criteria for mastery:	Four out of five opportunities
Final Goal:	The student will retell a grade level short story that has been read to him and include a beginning, middle, and end detail in four out of five opportunities.
How the skill will be measured:	Data collection

Main Idea and Details

Example 9

Prerequisite Skill: Important versus unimportant details

Step to Mastery: Determine important from unimportant details in a ___#___ sentence story

The skill to be worked on:	Determine important from unimportant details
How the student is expected to respond:	Will label
What material will be used:	Six-sentence story
How material will be presented:	Read aloud to student with text available
Cues/Prompts/Supports:	One visual cue
Criteria for mastery:	Three out of five opportunities
Final Goal: How the skill will be measured:	The student will label details as important or unimportant after listening to a six-sentence story while following along with one visual cue for three out of five opportunities. Data collection

Example 10

Prerequisite Skill: Identify main idea and supporting details

Steps to Mastery: Identify ___#___ details that support a given main idea in a (paragraph, story, poem, chapter, etc.)

The skill to be worked on:	Identify details that support a given main idea
How the student is expected to respond:	Will state
What material will be used:	Grade-level paragraph
How material will be presented:	Orally with text available
Cues/Prompts/Supports:	One verbal cue
Criteria for mastery:	Four out of five opportunities for two sessions
Final Goal:	The student will state two details that support a given main idea in a grade-level paragraph read to him while following along with one verbal cue in four out of five opportunities for two sessions.
How the skill will be measured:	Data collection

Critical Thinking

Example 11

Prerequisite Skill: Predict

Step to Mastery: Predict what will happen next in a _____ (story, chapter, etc.) and provide evidence for that prediction

The skill to be worked on:	Predicting
How the student is expected to respond:	Orally
What material will be used:	Six paragraphs from grade level material
How material will be presented:	Orally with text available
Cues/Prompts/Supports:	One verbal cue
Criteria for mastery:	80% accuracy for three sessions
Final Goal:	The student will predict what will happen next and provide evidence for that prediction when orally read six paragraphs from grade level text while following along with one verbal cue with 80% accuracy for three sessions.
How the skill will be measured:	Data collection

Example 12

Prerequisite Skill: Problem solve

Step to Mastery: Identify the problem in a situation

The skill to be worked on:	Identify the problem
How the student is expected to respond:	Will state
What material will be used:	Situation
How material will be presented:	Orally
Cues/Prompts/Supports:	None
Criteria for mastery:	70% of opportunities for three sessions
Final Goal:	The student will state the problem in an orally presented situation with 70% accuracy for three sessions.
How the skill will be measured:	Data collection

Example 13

Prerequisite Skill: Same/similar and different

Step to Mastery: State ___#___ similarities and ___#___ differences between two picture scenes

The skill to be worked on:	Similar and different
How the student is expected to respond:	Will state
What material will be used:	Picture scenes
How material will be presented:	Two picture scenes presented at same time
Cues/Prompts/Supports:	None
Criteria for master:	80% accuracy in three out of four opportunities
Final Goal:	The student will state three similarities and three differences when presented with two picture scenes with 80% accuracy in three out of four opportunities.
How the skill will be measured	Data collection

Pragmatics

Example 14

Prerequisite Skill: Request for object or action

Step to Mastery: Request desired _____ (object or action) using _____ (# words, whole sentence, etc.)

The skill to be worked on:	Request object
How the student is expected to respond:	Will verbally request
What material will be used:	Carrier phrase (I want ___)
How material will be presented:	Three picture choices
Cues/Prompts/Supports:	Carrier phrase (I want ___)
Criteria for mastery:	Four out of five opportunities for three sessions
Final Goal:	The student will request desired object given three picture choices using a carrier phrase (I want ___) in four out of five opportunities for three sessions.
How the skill will be measured:	Data collection

Example 15

Prerequisite Skill: Taking perspective of others

Step to Mastery: Explain two viewpoints/ideas for a given topic/situation

The skill to be worked on:	Perspective-taking
How the student is expected to respond:	Will verbally explain
What material will be used:	Topic or situation
How material will be presented:	Orally
Cues/Prompts/Supports:	One verbal cue
Criteria for mastery:	Four out of five opportunities for three sessions
Final Goal:	The student will verbally explain two viewpoints or ideas for an orally-presented topic or situation with one verbal cue for four out of five opportunities for three sessions.
How the skill will be measured:	Data collection

Syntax and Morphology

Example 16

Prerequisite Skill: Sentence construction

Step to Mastery: Use _____*_____ during _____ (structured conversation or unstructured conversation)

> *subject + object (Boy book)
>
> *subject + verb (Cat ran)
>
> *subject + verb + object (Boy read book)

The skill to be worked on:	Subject + verb + object (Boy read book)
How the student is expected to respond:	Orally with 3 word sentence in structured conversation
What material will be used:	Pictures
How material will be presented:	Student shown picture
Cues/Prompts/Supports:	None
Criteria for mastery:	60% accuracy for four sessions
Final Goal:	The student will use a three-word sentence consisting of subject + verb + object (boy read book) to describe pictures with 60% accuracy for four sessions.
How the skill will be measured:	Data collection and language sample

Example 17

Prerequisite Skill: Past tense

Steps to Mastery: Use _____ (regular or irregular) past tense:

- in words
- in sentences
- in structured conversation
- in unstructured conversation
- during academic instruction

The skill to be worked on:	Using regular past tense verbs
How the student is expected to respond:	Will orally use
What material will be used:	Pictures
How material will be presented:	Shown picture and asked to make a sentence
Cues/Prompts/Supports:	one visual cue
Criteria for mastery:	70% accuracy for four sessions
Final Goal:	The student will use regular past tense verbs in sentences when shown a picture with 1 visual cue with 70% accuracy for four sessions.
How the skill will be measured:	Data collection and language sample

Articulation and Phonological Processes

Example 18

Prerequisite Skill: /l/

Step to Mastery: Produce _____ (specify sounds) in _____

The skill to be worked on:	Production of /l/
How the student is expected to respond:	Orally produce
What material will be used:	Student-generated sentences
How material will be presented:	Orally
Cues/Prompts/Supports:	one visual cue
Criteria for mastery:	80% accuracy for three sessions
Final Goal:	The student will produce /l/ in sentences with 1 visual cue with 80% accuracy for three sessions.
How the skill will be measured:	Data collection

Example 19

Prerequisite Skill: Cluster reduction

Step to Mastery: Produce two sounds for each blend in _____

The skill to be worked on:	Production of blends
How the student is expected to respond:	Orally produce
What material will be used:	Student-generated sentences
How material will be presented:	Orally
Cues/Prompts/Supports:	Picture prompt
Criteria for mastery:	70% accuracy for four sessions
Final Goal:	The student will produce two sounds for each blend in sentences with a picture prompt with 70% accuracy for four sessions.
How the skill will be measured:	Data collection

APPENDIX 4–1
Goal Writing Worksheet

Prerequisite Skill: _____

Step to Mastery: _____

The skill to be worked on:	
How the student is expected to respond:	
What material will be used:	
How material will be presented:	
Cues/Prompts/Supports:	
Criteria for mastery:	
Final Goal:	
How the skill will be measured:	

References

American Speech-Language-Hearing Association (ASHA). (2010). *Roles and responsibilities of speech-language pathologists in schools* [Professional issues statement]. Retrieved from http://www.asha.org/policy

American Speech-Language-Hearing Association (ASHA). (2010). *Components of social communication (Pragmatics).* Retrieved from http://www.asha.org/Practice-Portal/

American Speech-Language-Hearing Association (ASHA). (2001). *Roles and responsibilities of speech-language pathologists with respect to reading and writing in children and adolescents* [Guidelines]. Retrieved from http://www.asha.org/policy

American Speech-Language-Hearing Association (ASHA). (2014). *Social language use (Pragmatics).* Retrieved from http://www.asha.org/public/speech/development/Pragmatics/

American Speech-Language-Hearing Association (ASHA). (2014). *Typical speech and language development.* Retrieved from http://www.asha.org/public/speech/development/

Banotai, A. (2010, July 12). Evidence-based vocabulary instruction: Strategies for word learning and comprehension. *Advance for Speech and Hearing, 20(4),* p. 9. Retrieved from http://speech-language-pathology-audiology.advanceweb.com/Archives/

Beck, I. L., Kucan, L., & McKeown, M. G. (2013). *Bringing words to life: Robust vocabulary instruction* (2nd ed.). New York, NY: The Guilford Press.

Bloom, L., Merkin, S., & Wootten, J. (1982). "Wh"-Questions: Linguistic factors that contribute to the sequence of acquisition. *Child Development, 53(4),* 1084–1092. doi: 10.2307/1129150

Bowen, C. (n.d.). *Cycles Phonological Pattern Approach (CPPA).* Retrieved from http://www.speech-language-therapy.com

Bowen, C. (2012). *Table 2: Phonological processes.* Retrieved from http://speech-language-therapy.com

Bowen, C. (2013). *Brown's stages of syntactic and morphological development.* Retrieved from http://speech-language-therapy.com

Brandone, A .C., Salkind, S. J., Golinkoff, R. M., & Hirsch-Pasek, K. (2006). Language development. In G. C. Bear & K. M. Minke (Eds.), *Children's needs III: Development, prevention, and intervention* (pp. 499–514). Bethesda, MD: National Association of School Psychologists

Byrne, J. (2005). *The Barrett taxonomy of cognitive and affective dimensions of reading comprehension.* Retrieved from http://joebyrne.net/Curriculum/barrett.pdf

Center for Speech and Language Pathology. (n.d). *Early morphological development.* Retrieved from http://www.speechtherapyct.com/whats_new/Early%20Morphological%20Development.pdf

Center for Speech and Language Pathology. (2014). Early morphological development [Article]. Retrieved from http://www.speechtherapyct.com/whatsnew.htm

Conrad-Curry, D. (2013). Retell, recount, summarize? A common core shift from kindergarten to fourth grade [Blog post]. Retrieved from http://partnerinedu.com/2013/01/29/retell-or-recount-the-common-core-shift-from-1st-grade-to-2nd-grade/

Dawson, J. I., Stout, C. E., & Eyer, J. A. (2003). *Structured photographic expressive language test* [Manual] (3rd ed.). DeKalb, IL: Janelle.

Early Childhood Leadership Institute. (2012). *District of Columbia Common Core Early Learning Standards.* Retrieved from Office of the State Superintendent of Education: http://osse.dc.gov/publication/district-columbia-common-core-aligned-early-learning-standards

Ehren, B. (2002). Vocabulary intervention to improve reading comprehension for students with learning disabilities. *Perspectives on Language Learning and Education, 9,* 12–18. doi:10.1044/lle9.3.12

Gard, A., Gilman, L., & Gorman, J. (1993). *Speech and language development chart* (2nd ed.). Austin, TX: Pro-Ed

Georgia Department of Early Care and Learning. (2015). *Georgia Early Learning and Development Standards (GELDS).* Retrieved from http://gelds.decal.ga.gov/Default.aspx

Goldman, R., & Fristoe, M. (2000). *Goldman-Fristoe Test of Articulation 2nd edition* [Manual]. Circle Pines, MN: American Guidance Service.

Hodson, B. W. (2011). Enhancing phonological patterns of young children with highly unintelligible speech. *The ASHA Leader, April 5, 2011.* Retrieved from http://www.asha.org/Publications/

Hutton, T. L. (2008). Three tiers of vocabulary and education. *Super Duper® Handy Handouts!™ Number 182.* Retrieved from http://www.superduperinc.com

Kansas State Department of Education. (2014). *Early Learning Standards 2013 Revision.* Retrieved from Kansas State Department of Education: http://www.ksde.org

Klein, E. S. (1996). Phonological/traditional approaches to articulation therapy: A retrospective group comparison. *Language, Speech, and Hearing Services in Schools, 27,* 314–323. doi:10.1044/0161-1461.2704.314

Loraine, S. (2008). Vocabulary development. *Super Duper® Handy Handouts!™ Number 149.* Retrieved from http://www.superduperinc.com

Louisiana Department of Education. (2013). *Louisiana's birth to five early learning and development standards (ELDS).* Retrieved from Louisiana Department of Education: https://www.louisianabelieves.com

Mannheim, J. K. (2012). *Preschooler development.* Bethesda, MD: U.S. National Library of Medicine. Retrieved from http://www.nlm.nih.gov/medlineplus/ency/article/002013.htm

Marzano, R. J. (2004). *Building background knowledge for academic achievement: Research on what works in schools.* Alexandria, VA: Association for Supervision and Curriculum Development

Montgomery, J. K. (2007). *The bridge of vocabulary: Evidence-based activities for academic success.* Minneapolis,MN: NCS Pearson.

Morris, P. (n.d). Developmental hierarchy for negation [Blog post]. Retrieved from http://freelanguagestuff.com/negation/

National Dissemination Center for Children with Disabilities [NICHCY]. (2010). *Annual goals.* Retrieved from http://nichcy.org/schoolage/iep/iepcontents/goals

National Governors Association Center for Best Practices [NGA] & Council of Chief State School Officers [CCSS]. (2010). *Common Core State Standards.* Retrieved from http://www.corestandards.org

National Reading Technical Assistance Center [NRTAC]. (2010). *A review of the current research on vocabulary instruction.* Retrieved from U.S. Department of Education: http://www.ed.gov/programs/readingfirst/support/index.html

North Carolina Foundations Task Force. (2013). *North Carolina foundations for early learning and development.* Retrieved from Public Schools of North Carolina Office of Early Learning: http://www.ncpublicschools.org/earlylearning/

Office of Head Start. (2015). *Head Start early learning outcomes framework: Ages birth to five.* Retrieved from Early Childhood Learning & Knowledge Center (ECLKC): http://eclkc.ohs.acf.hhs.gov/hslc

PLD Learning Resources. (2014). *Skill set 1: Oral language; Semantic development milestones.* Retrieved from www.pld-literacy.org/semantic-development-milestones-fact-sheet.html

Rebhorn, T. (2009). Developing your child's IEP. *A Parent's Guide, 12,* 1–28. Retrieved from http://nichcy.org/publications/pa12

Rhode Island Department of Education. (2015). *Rhode Island early learning and development standards.* Retrieved from http://rields.com/

Robinson, L., & Westby, C. (2009). Social or academic language intervention? You don't have to choose. *Perspectives on Language Learning and Education, 16,* 42–47. doi:10.1044/lle16.2.42

Rose, D., & Gravel, J. (2010). *Technology and learning meeting special student's needs.* Wakefield, MA: National Center on Universal Design for Learning. Retrieved from http://www.udlcenter.org/sites/udlcenter.org/files/TechnologyandLearniing.pdf

Roth, F. P. (2002). Vocabulary instruction for young children with language impairments. *Perspectives on Language Learning and Education, 9,* 3–7. doi:10.1044/lle9.3.3

Rowland, C. F., Pine, J. M., Lieven, E. V., & Theaksston, A. L. (2003). Determinants of acquisition order in wh-questions: Re-evaluating the role of caregiver speech. *Journal of Child Language. 30,* 609–635.

Sander, E. K. (1972). When are speech sounds learned? *Journal of Speech and Hearing Disorders, 37,* 55–63. doi:10.1044/jshd.3701.55

Sax, N., & Weston, E. (2007). *Language development milestones.* Retrieved from http://www.rehabmed.ualberta.ca/spa/phonology/milestones.pdf

Smit, A. B., Hand, L., Freilinger, J. J., Bernthal, J. E., & Bird, A. (1990). The Iowa articulation norms projects and its Nebraska replication. *Journal of Speech and Hearing Disorders, 55,* 779–798. doi:10.1044/jshd.5504.779

Spielvogle, K. (n.d.). Articulation vs. phonology, Van Riper vs. Hodson? What's a busy therapist to do? *Super Duper® Handy Handouts!™ Number 45* Retrieved from http://www.superduperinc.com

Spivey, B. L. (2006). How to help your child understand and produce "Wh" questions. *Super Duper® Handy Handouts!™ Number 110* Retrieved from http://www.superduperinc.com

Stewart, R. (n.d.). *Should we insist on eye contact with people who have autism spectrum disorders?* Retrieved from http://autism-help.org/communication-eye-contact.htm

Tennessee Department of Education. (2013). *Early Learning Developmental Standards (TN-ELDS).* Retrieved from Tennessee Department of Education: http://tn.gov/education

Thompson, R. M. (n.d) Saying no without offending. In *Interaction and English grammar.* Retrieved from http://www.clas.ufl.edu/users/rthompso/interactioncontents.html

U.S. Department of Education. (2004). *Individuals with Disabilities Education Act (IDEA).* Retrieved from http://idea.ed.gov/

U.S. Department of Education. (2007). *Modified academic achievement standards* [non-regulatory guidance draft]. Washington, DC: Author. Retrieved from http://www.ed.gov/policy/speced/guid/nclb/twopercent.doc

Van Riper, C. (1978). *Speech correction: Principles and methods* (6th ed.). Englewood Cliffs, NJ: Prentice-Hall

Wiig, E., Secord, W. A., & Semel, E. (2004). *Clinical evaluation of language fundamentals preschool* (2nd ed.). San Antonio, TX: Harcourt Assessment.

Winner, M. G. (2007). *Thinking about YOU, thinking about ME* (2nd ed.). San Jose, CA: Think Social.

Winner, M. G. (2008). *Think social! A social thinking curriculum for school-age students.* San Jose, CA: Think Social.

Winner, M. G., & Crooke, P.J. (2009). Social Thinking®: A developmental treatment approach for students with social learning/social pragmatic challenges. *Perspectives on Language Learning and Education, 16*(2), 62–69. Retrieved from http://www.socialthinking.com/what-is-social-thinking/overview-of-social-thinking

Wright, P., & Wright, P. (2006). *Wrightslaw: From emotions to advocacy* (2nd ed., excerpted from Chapter 12). Hartfield, VA: Harbor House Law Press. Retrieved from http://www.wrightslaw.com/bks/feta2/ch12.ieps.pdf

Index

Note: Page numbers in **bold** reference non-text material.